# EPILEPSY

## QUESTIONS AND ANSWERS

**MERIT PUBLISHING INTERNATIONAL**

*European address:*
35 Winchester Street
Basingstoke
Hampshire RG21 7EE
England

*North American address:*
8260 NW 49th Manor
Pine Grove, Coral Springs
Florida 33067
U.S.A.

ISBN 1 873413 80 7 (English)
ISBN 1 873413 51 3 (French)

J W SANDER

Y M HART

**merit**
PUBLISHING
INTERNATIONAL

# ACKNOWLEDGEMENTS

We would like to express our thanks to the many colleagues who have given us advice and encouragement. We are particularly grateful to Dr Raymond Ali, Dr John Duncan, Dr David Fish, Dr Li Li Min, and Dr Sanjay Sisodiya for their helpful comments and for supplying many of the illustrations. We would like to thank the Information and Education Services Department of the National Society for Epilepsy for supplying us with the questions shown in Chapter 13.

We are indebted to Professor Simon Shorvon and Professor Frederick Andermann for their guidance, teaching and encouragement. Last, but by no means least, we would like to thank all the people with epilepsy we have met and from whom we have learned so much. This book would not have been possible without their help, and we dedicate it to them.


J W Sander, Y M Hart

# CONTENTS

# INTRODUCTION

Epilepsy is a common medical condition, with a lifetime incidence estimated at 2-5%. The majority of patients diagnosed as having epilepsy have only a few seizures, usually each lasting only minutes, and yet the implications of the diagnosis are often considerable, particularly in the areas of employment, education and leisure. Apart from the limitations imposed by the risk of a seizure itself, epilepsy has long been beset by myths and negative conceptions, even among the medical profession, which until recently considered epilepsy to be a lifelong condition with a uniformly poor prognosis.

This book has been written for general physicians, general practitioners, neurologists in training, and medical students, to provide a concise core of background information on the nature, causes, and treatment of epilepsy, and to supply answers to some of the questions most commonly asked regarding these issues. It is not intended to supplant standard textbooks of epilepsy, which are recommended for further reading and reference. A basic knowledge of neuroanatomy and physiology has been assumed.

The publication is divided into thirteen chapters. The first five describe the epidemiology, nature and characteristics of epilepsy and other seizure disorders. Chapter six addresses the question of the diagnosis of epilepsy and the investigations which may be required to confirm diagnosis, classify the type of epilepsy and evaluate the underlying cause. The next two chapters deal with the types of medical and surgical treatment currently available and their indications. Women with epilepsy pose some specific problems such as the management of epilepsy during pregnancy, the issue of teratogenicity associated with antiepileptic drugs, menstruation and contraception, and these are dealt with in chapter nine. The psychiatric aspects of epilepsy, and the issues of genetic counselling in epilepsy are addressed in the next two chapters. Chapter twelve deals with the issues of leisure and work, while the final chapter is a selection of questions frequently asked by people with epilepsy. A reading list and the addresses of epilepsy organisations are also provided in the appendices.

Epilepsy poses a number of peculiar problems. Unlike most ailments, it is episodic: in between seizures, physical examination and laboratory investigation of patients may be perfectly normal. The diagnosis is, therefore, essentially clinical, relying on the patient's account and those of eye-witnesses, and it may be difficult to differentiate from the myriad of other episodic conditions capable of causing transient impairment of consciousness or other symptoms. Because of the potential impact on the patient's life, however, it is imperative that the correct diagnosis be reached, and that optimum treatment and advice be given.

Although we have tried to ensure that the information contained in this book, particularly pertaining to drugs, is accurate, drug information may change from time to time and clinicians are advised to consult manufacturers' information sheets before prescribing drugs.

# E PILEPSY

## QUESTIONS AND ANSWERS

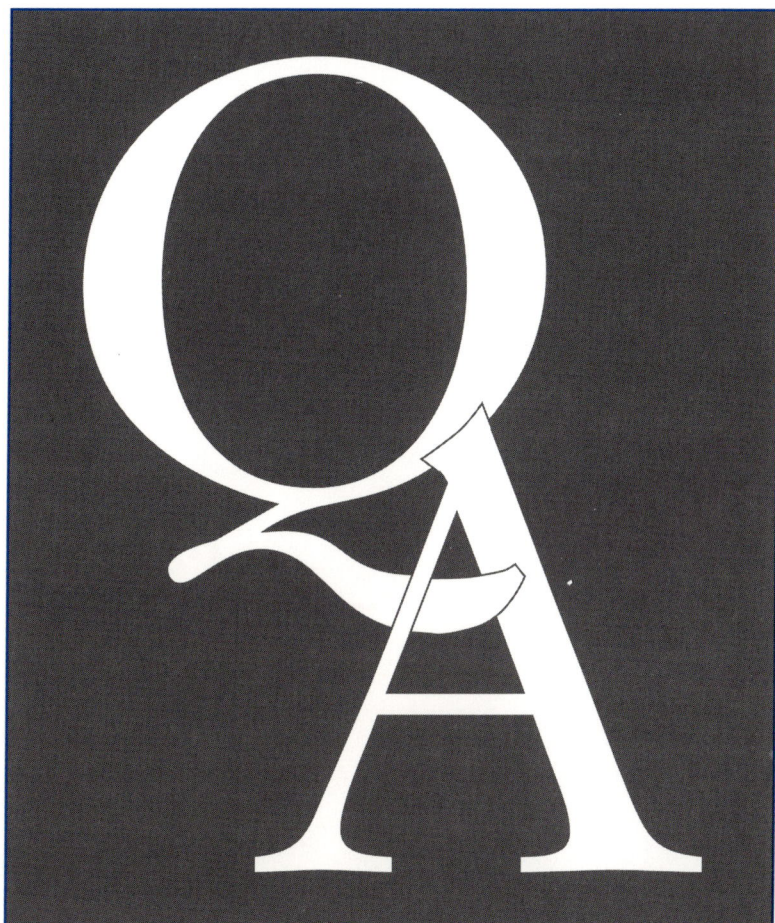

J W SANDER

Y M HART

merit
PUBLISHING
INTERNATIONAL

# CHAPTER 1

## WHAT IS EPILEPSY?

*Epilepsy is one of the most common neurological conditions, occurring in the range of 0.5 - 1.0% of the general population in developed countries.* It is also one of the oldest recorded medical conditions, having been accurately described by Hippocrates more than 2000 years ago. The word "epilepsy" is derived from a Greek term, meaning to possess, to take hold of, to grab or to seize. To the ancient Greeks, epilepsy was a miraculous phenomenon; they considered that only the gods could knock someone down, strip their reason, make their body thrash around uncontrollably, and afterwards bring them around without apparent ill-effect.

**a common neurological condition**

The first modern definition of epilepsy was given by Hughlings Jackson in the second half of the 19th century. He defined it as *"the occasional, sudden, excessive, rapid and local discharge of grey matter"*, and this definition is among those used today, although it should be pointed out that discharges detected electrographically are not generally considered to be clinical seizures unless they are accompanied by changes which can be detected either by the patient or an observer. An operational definition of epilepsy often used currently is *"the occurrence of transient paroxysms of excessive or uncontrolled discharges of neurons, which may be caused by a number of different aetiologies, leading to epileptic seizures"*. The actual form which an epileptic seizure takes depends on the location of the initial epileptic discharge and its spread.

**excessive discharges of neurons**

*It is necessary for seizures to be recurrent and unprovoked to constitute epilepsy*; by definition a single attack is not considered sufficient to make this diagnosis, even though most people having one seizure will have further attacks. Epileptic seizures occurring only in association with precipitants or trigger factors are termed acute symptomatic or situation-related seizures: even if recurrent, they are not usually considered as "epilepsy". Such precipitants include fever in young children, sleep deprivation, strokes, metabolic imbalance, alcohol or drug abuse, acute head trauma, and the consumption of known epileptogenic drugs.

**seizures must be recurrent**

*It should be stressed that seizures are a symptom of disease, rather than a single well-defined illness*. The term "epilepsy" is thus loosely applied

**seizures are a symptom of disease**

to a number of seizure disorders that have in common only a tendency for the patient to have recurrent epileptic attacks, and it has been argued that "the epilepsies" is a more appropriate term than "epilepsy". There are a number of conditions presenting with epileptic seizures which are associated with well-defined clinical and electrophysiological characteristics that allow them to be grouped into specific epileptic syndromes, but a large number of people developing seizures cannot be grouped into such categories.

### 1.1 What is an epileptic seizure?

**a discernible event**  *An epileptic seizure* (also termed "ictus" or "ictal event") *is a transient paroxysm of excessive discharges of neurons in the cerebral cortex causing an event which is discernible to the person experiencing the seizure or an observer.*  The clinical manifestations of seizures may take many different forms, varying from patient to patient and reflecting the functions of the cortical tissues in which the excessive discharge arises and to which it spreads.

**awareness may be impaired**  *A seizure is a stereotyped event in which an individual's awareness of his surroundings may be impaired and behaviour altered.*  Motor signs, sensory or psychic experiences, autonomic disturbances and negative neurological phenomena (such as speech arrest or loss of muscle tone) may also occur in combination or isolation, sometimes in a progressive manner.  **sudden onset**  *Epileptic seizures frequently have a sudden onset and usually cease spontaneously.*  They are commonly brief, lasting from seconds to minutes, and are often followed by a period of drowsiness and confusion **cease spontaneously**  (the post-ictal period).

The word seizure is also occasionally used for other transient non-epileptic events such as syncope, psychogenic attacks, night terrors, and temper tantrums, and it is thus advisable to use the term "epileptic seizure" when **terms used by the public**  referring to an epileptic event. *Many different terms are used by the public to describe epileptic seizures*; some of the more frequently used are fits, spells, funny turns, attacks, and blackouts.

# CHAPTER 2

## THE CLASSIFICATION OF EPILEPTIC SEIZURES AND SYNDROMES

### 2.1 How are epileptic seizures classified?

*There are several ways in which epileptic seizures may be classified.* These include classification by underlying aetiology, by age at onset, by the topographic location of the abnormal discharge, by the clinical manifestations, by the findings on the electroencephalogram (EEG), or by the types of seizures themselves. The question of classification is controversial and there is no universal agreement as to the most appropriate method. However, *the most commonly used classification of epileptic seizures is the International Seizure Classification proposed by the International League against Epilepsy (ILAE)*, which is based on the clinical and electroencephalographic manifestations of a seizure (Table 1). It divides epileptic seizures into two main groups according to the source of the primary epileptic discharge: those originating from localised cortical areas, the epileptic focus or foci (partial seizures) and those characterised by synchronous discharges over both hemispheres (generalised seizures). It does not take into account the background aetiology or any anatomic feature. In addition, there is a group of seizures which are deemed "unclassifiable" even after extensive investigation, such as may occur in patients with infrequent and unwitnessed events.

**classification of epileptic seizures**

**International League against Epilepsy**

### 2.2 What are partial seizures?

*Partial or focal seizures arise from an epileptic focus, that is, a localised region of cerebral cortex in which the excessive discharge of neurons originates.* The clinical manifestations of a partial seizure depend on the position of the focus in the cerebral cortex, whether the discharge remains localised or spreads, and if it spreads, the cortical pathways involved. *The most common sites of origin of epileptic seizures are the temporal lobes*. Seizures arising from the frontal lobes are also not uncommon. Less frequently the site of origin of the seizure is found in the parietal or occipital regions.

**partial seizures arise from a localised region**

**most common sites are the temporal lobes**

**Table 1.** *International Classification of Epileptic Seizures.*

---

**I. PARTIAL SEIZURES** (seizures beginning locally)
**A.** Simple partial seizures (consciousness not impaired)
1. With motor symptoms
2. With somatosensory or special sensory symptoms
3. With autonomic symptoms
4. With psychic symptoms
**B.** Complex partial seizures (with impairment of consciousness)
1. Beginning as simple partial seizures and progressing to
   impairment of consciousness
a. With no other features
b. With features as in A.1-4
c. With automatisms
2. With impairment of consciousness at onset
a. With no other features
b. With features as in A.1-4
c. With automatisms
**C.** Partial seizures secondarily generalised

**II. GENERALISED SEIZURES**
(Bilaterally symmetrical and without focal onset)
**A.** 1. Absence seizures
   2. Atypical absence seizures
**B.** Myoclonic seizures
**C.** Clonic seizures
**D.** Tonic seizures
**E.** Tonic clonic seizures
**F.** Atonic seizures

**III. UNCLASSIFIED EPILEPTIC SEIZURES**
(inadequate or incomplete data)

Epilepsia 1981, 22:489-501

---

**nature of the seizure** The partial nature of the seizure and the location of the focus can often be identified from the clinical signs present either during or after the seizure. The "aura" or warning occurring prior to a seizure experienced by some patients usually reflects the function of that part of the cerebral cortex in which the epileptic discharge initially occurs. If the epileptic discharge remains localised it is likely that the patient will remain aware throughout the attack, as the rest of the cortex continues to function normally. If it spreads to the limbic system consciousness may be altered, and if further spread occurs a generalised tonic clonic seizure (secondarily generalised seizure) may ensue. If, however, the discharge starts in the limbic system, consciousness may be impaired from the onset of the seizure and again, a generalised tonic clonic convulsion may follow. Another sign which indicates the partial nature of a seizure is the occurrence of post-ictal focal neurological deficits. For example, a patient may experience a transient post-ictal hemiparesis (Todd's paresis), amaurosis, or aphasia. *The EEG tracing recorded from the scalp can also sometimes be useful in identifying the location of the focus* (see Figure 1). However, in patients in whom the site of origin is remote from the surface electrodes, or in whom generalisation occurs very quickly, this may not be possible. In these cases, intracranial (or depth) EEG recording may be helpful if surgery is being considered.

**EEG is also useful in identification of focus**

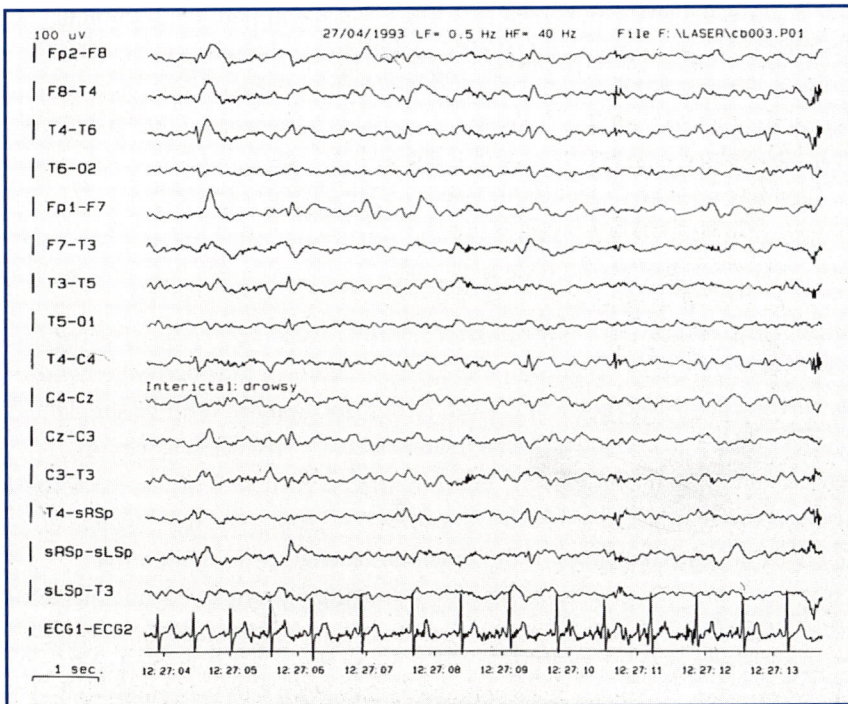

100 uV        27/04/1993 LF= 0.5 Hz HF= 40 Hz        File F: \LASER\cD003.P01
Fp2-F8
F8-T4
T4-T6
T6-O2
Fp1-F7
F7-T3
T3-T5
T5-O1
T4-C4
C4-Cz       Interictal: drowsy
Cz-C3
C3-T3
T4-sRSp
sRSp-sLSp
sLSp-T3
ECG1-ECG2

1 sec.  12:27:04  12:27:05  12:27:06  12:27:07  12:27:08  12:27:09  12:27:10  12:27:11  12:27:12  12:27:13

**Figure 1.** *EEG showing interictal focal epileptic activity (Courtesy of Dr David Fish).*

### 2.3 How are partial seizures sub-divided ?

Partial seizures are sub-divided into three groups: simple partial, complex partial, and partial with secondary generalisation.

### Simple partial seizures

**consciousness is fully preserved**

*Simple partial seizures are epileptic events in which consciousness is fully preserved, and in which the discharge usually remains localised.* Isolated simple partial seizures are relatively rare as they usually progress to other forms of partial seizures. Simple partial seizures are more common in patients with seizures starting late in life rather than in childhood, and almost invariably indicate the presence of a structural lesion involving the cortex. The precise clinical manifestations of a simple partial seizure depend on the cortical area in which the discharge occurs and may vary widely from patient to patient, but will usually assume the same form in one patient. Examples of such manifestations include involuntary localised motor disturbances, which may be tonic or clonic in nature, autonomic disturbances, and sensory or psychic experiences. Simple partial seizures usually start suddenly and are brief, unless progression occurs. If seizure spread occurs so that consciousness is impaired, the seizure evolves into a complex partial seizure. If it progresses further and a convulsive seizure occurs, it is termed a secondarily generalised seizure. When such progression occurs, the early part of the seizure, in which consciousness is preserved, is called the aura or warning.

**involvement of body parts**

*Motor disturbances in simple partial seizures may involve any part of the body*, although most commonly the face and limbs, particularly the hands, are involved. A well-known, though rather uncommon, form of simple partial motor seizure is the "Jacksonian seizure". This starts as clonic jerking in one part of the body, often in a hand, which slowly spreads to contiguous muscle groups in the so-called "Jacksonian march", which parallels the slow progress of the epileptic discharge along the motor cortex. Occasionally, simple partial seizures may be followed by transient weakness or even paralysis of the muscle groups involved in the seizure (Todd's paresis).

Simple partial seizures may sometimes involve auditory, olfactory or visual hallucinations which may be confounded with psychotic symptomatology. In favour of an epileptic nature for hallucinations are the stereotyped nature of the attack and the fact that the patient is usually aware that the hallucinations are not real. In schizophrenia, in contrast, stereotyping of the hallucinations is absent and the patient does not have insight.

It is rather unusual for simple partial seizures to occur as the sole manifestation of epilepsy, although it may be that, because they cause little or no disability, they occur more frequently than is recognised. *The development of simple partial seizures indicates the need to search for the underlying aetiology, and in particular to rule out an expanding intracerebral lesion.*

**search for underlying aetiology**

## Complex partial seizures

*Complex partial seizures*, one of the most common types of seizure, may have similar characteristics to simple partial seizures, but *by definition always involve an impairment of consciousness*. They are often termed "psychomotor seizures". Another term sometimes used for complex partial seizures, mainly in medical circles, is "temporal lobe epilepsy". However, it should be stressed that although the majority of complex partial seizures originate in the temporal lobes, many complex partial seizures originate elsewhere, particularly in the frontal lobes.

**impairment of consciousness**

Complex partial seizures may start as a simple partial seizure and then progress, or the patient may have alteration of consciousness from the onset. If the attack begins as a simple partial seizure, this may act as a warning (or "aura") to the patient that a seizure is about to start.

*It is not uncommon for complex partial seizures to present as altered or "automatic" behaviour.* The patient may pluck at his or her clothes, fiddle with various objects and act in a confused manner. Lip-smacking or chewing movements, grimacing, undressing, and the carrying out of purposeless activities or of aimless wandering may occur on their own or in different combinations. Complex partial seizures are usually followed by confusion in the post-ictal period; alternatively they may progress to a secondarily generalised seizure.

**altered or "automatic" behaviour**

Automatic behaviour may occur either as an ictal phenomenon or in the post-ictal period. Ictal automatisms may be either spontaneous or reactive, the former type being stereotyped, so that they usually assume the same form in each seizure. They commonly involve oroalimentary automatisms (lip-smacking, swallowing and chewing), mimetic automatisms (grimacing and other facial expressions), gestural automatisms (fiddling with clothes, undressing, scratching, rearranging objects), ambulatory automatisms (walking or running) and verbal automatisms (uttering names or phrases). Spontaneous sexual automatisms are much rarer than the above and usually involve masturbation.

**determined by environmental circumstances**

*Reactive automatisms are not stereotyped, but are usually determined by environmental circumstances.* They generally occur when a patient has a seizure whilst a task is being carried out, and is able to carry on with very few outward signs of a seizure in progression. The tasks are usually simple, although on occasion more complex tasks may be performed. In the latter situation, however, inappropriate response is more common.

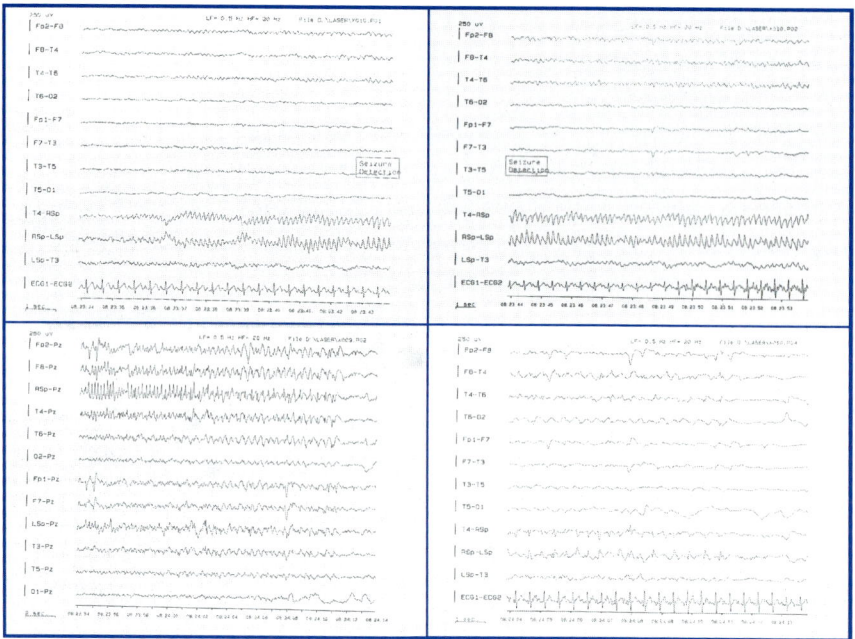

**Figure 2.** *EEG showing progression of partial seizure originating in the right temporal lobe. (Courtesy of Dr David Fish).*

### Secondarily generalised seizures

**tonic clonic convulsion**

*Secondarily generalised attacks are partial seizures, either simple or complex, in which the epileptic discharge spreads to both cerebral hemispheres, so that a generalised seizure, usually a tonic clonic convulsion, ensues.* The patient may have an aura, but this is not always the case. The spread of the discharge can occur so quickly that no features of the localised onset are apparent to the patient or to an observer, and in that case only an EEG can demonstrate the partial nature of the seizure (Figure 2). On rare occasions a secondarily generalised seizure may take the form of a tonic, atonic or unilateral tonic clonic seizure.

### 2.4 What are generalised seizures?

*Generalised seizures are characterised by the simultaneous involvement of the whole cortex at the onset of the seizure*. This can usually be demonstrated by an EEG. Patients experiencing generalised seizures lose consciousness at the beginning of the seizure, so that there is no warning. There are various types of generalised seizures (see Table 1). Among the most common generalised epileptic attacks are generalised tonic clonic seizures, absence seizures, myoclonic, tonic, and atonic seizures.

**involvement of the whole cortex**

### Generalised tonic clonic seizures

*Generalised tonic clonic convulsions, or convulsive seizures, are common. They used to be called "grand mal" attacks, and this term is still widely used*. In this type of seizure, there is no warning whatsoever, but the patient may experience a prodrome, sometimes lasting hours, of general malaise. At the onset of the seizure (the tonic phase), the patient becomes stiff, often crying out. The tongue may also be bitten during this phase. Apnoea occurs, and the patient becomes cyanosed. The heart rate and blood pressure increase. The patient falls, breathing becomes laboured, salivation occurs, and clonic movements, usually involving all four limbs, develop (the clonic phase). This phase consist of intermittent clonic movements involving most muscles, followed by brief periods of muscle relaxation. The latter gradually become longer and eventually the clonic movements cease altogether, marking the end of the seizure. Incontinence commonly occurs at the end of the clonic phase. The convulsion usually ceases after a few minutes and is followed by a post-ictal period of drowsiness, confusion, headache and sleep. *It is not uncommon for people to fall deeply asleep after a convulsion and this may sometimes be misinterpreted as unconsciousness*. When they wake up they will be unaware of what has happened, will often feel lethargic, and may complain of generalised muscle aches due to the strenuous muscle activity of the clonic phase.

**convulsive seizures are common**

**deep sleep after a convulsion**

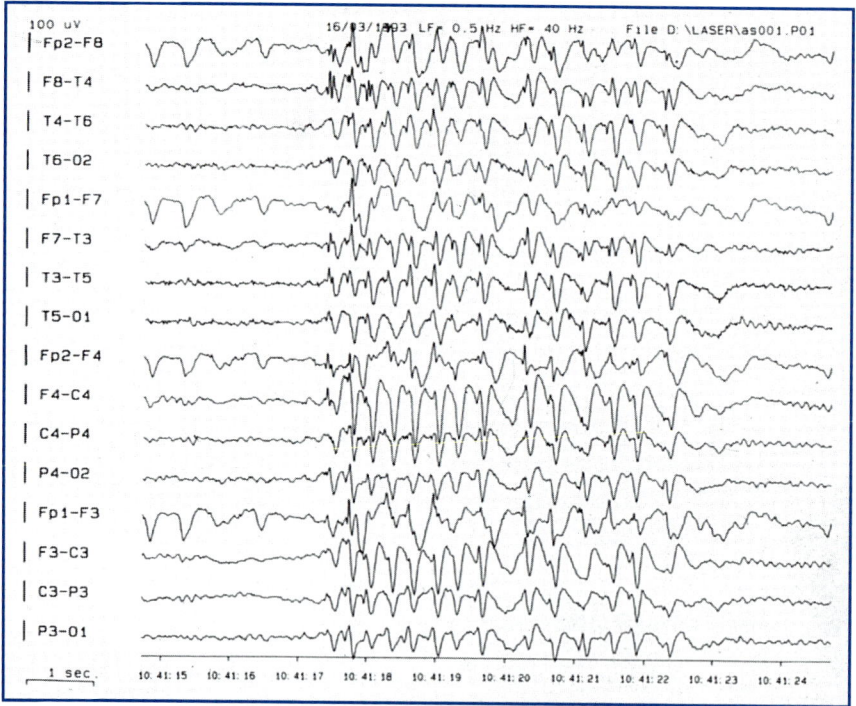

**Figure 3.** *EEG showing 3 per second spike and wave discharges in primary generalised epilepsy. (Courtesy of Dr Li Li Min).*

## Absence seizures

*Typical absence attacks*, also known as "petit mal", are a much rarer form of generalised seizure. *They occur almost exclusively in childhood and early adolescence*. The child suddenly appears blank and stares: fluttering of the eyelids, swallowing, and flopping of the head may occur. The attacks last only a few seconds and often pass unrecognised. Not infrequently, they are diagnosed only when learning difficulties at school are investigated in a child who has problems in concentrating due to frequent absence attacks. Absence attacks are associated with a characteristic EEG pattern, the so-called 3 per second generalised spike-and-wave discharges (Figure 3). They may be precipitated by hyperventilation, which is a useful diagnostic manoeuvre.

## Myoclonic seizures

*Myoclonic seizures are abrupt, very brief, involuntary flexion movements which may involve the whole body, or part of it, for example the arms or head.*

They occur most commonly in the morning, shortly after waking. They may sometimes cause the patient to fall, but recovery is immediate. The majority of myoclonic seizures occur in relatively benign seizure conditions but sometimes they herald more severe disorders. Not all myoclonus is the result of epilepsy: non-epileptic myoclonic jerks occur in a variety of other neurological conditions including lesions of the brainstem and spinal cord. Myoclonus is usually termed "epileptic" if it occurs in the context of a seizure disorder without evidence of encephalopathy, at least initially, and "symptomatic" if it accompanies an encephalopathy which is the predominant feature. Examples of conditions often accompanied by myoclonus are acute cerebral hypoxia or ischaemia, and degenerative brain diseases such as Creutzfeld-Jakob disease. In addition, *myoclonic seizures may also occur in healthy people*, particularly when they are just going off to sleep (hypnic jerk, hypnogogic myoclonus, or nocturnal start), and are then considered to be a normal physiological phenomenon.

**abrupt, brief, involuntary flexion movements**

**may occur in healthy people**

### Atonic and tonic seizures

*These types of generalised attacks are very rare, accounting for less than 1% of the epileptic attacks seen in the general population.* They usually occur during the course of some forms of severe epilepsy, often starting in early childhood, such as the Lennox-Gastaut syndrome or myoclonic astatic epilepsy. Atonic seizures (sometimes called akinetic attacks or drop attacks) involve a sudden loss of tone in the postural muscles, and the patient falls to the ground. There are no convulsive movements. Recovery is rapid, with no perceptible post-ictal symptomatology. During tonic seizures, there is a sudden increase in the muscle tone of the body and the patient becomes rigid, usually falling backwards onto the ground. Again, recovery is generally rapid. *Tonic and atonic attacks are often accompanied by severe injury.*

**less than 1% of epileptic attacks**

### 2.5 How are the epileptic syndromes classified?

*In addition to classifying epileptic seizures by type, a number of distinctive epileptic syndromes have been recognised* (a syndrome being a specific constellation of symptoms and signs). In the case of epilepsy, syndromes are usually defined by the features of the seizures, the presence of characteristic structural lesions, the age of onset of the condition, the presence of a family history, and by typical changes in the EEG. It is

**distinctive epileptic syndromes**

important to try to categorise epilepsies according to the syndromic classification if possible, since this may have implications both for prognosis and treatment;  in addition, it may prove possible to anticipate particular complications of certain syndromes.  However, not all patients with chronic seizure disorders fit into such a classification.

**classification scheme**

*A classification scheme for epileptic syndromes and related disorders proposed by the ILAE, although controversial* and with a number of limitations, *is currently used in most tertiary referral centres* (see Table 2). It classifies epileptic syndromes into four groups:  localisation-related (partial or focal), generalised, undetermined and special syndromes. Within these groups the syndromes are further divided into three sub-groups:  primary or idiopathic, secondary or symptomatic, and cryptogenic. When epileptic seizures are the only symptom of an inherited or genetic

**"idiopathic" refers to an inherited disorder**

disorder, the syndrome is termed primary;  when they occur as symptoms of a condition associated with structural brain lesions, the syndrome is termed symptomatic or secondary, and when the aetiology of the condition is unknown the term cryptogenic is used.  The terms "idiopathic" and "cryptogenic" are sometimes used interchangeably for disorders in which the specific aetiology has not been identified.  *This should, however, be avoided, and the term "idiopathic" reserved for those syndromes which are presumed to be inherited.*

**Table 2.** *International Classification of Epilepsies, Epileptic Syndromes, and related disorders.*

---

### 1. LOCALISATION-RELATED (FOCAL, LOCAL, PARTIAL)
Idiopathic (primary)
**1.1**     Benign childhood epilepsy with centro-temporal spikes
Childhood epilepsy with occipital paroxysms
Primary reading epilepsy

Symptomatic (secondary)
**1.2**     Temporal lobe epilepsies
Frontal lobe epilepsies
Parietal lobe epilepsies
Occipital lobe epilepsies
Chronic progressive epilepsia partialis continua of childhood
Syndromes characterised by seizures with specific modes of precipitation

---

continued on next page

Cryptogenic

**1.3**    defined by:

Seizure type

Clinical features

Aetiology

Anatomical localisation

## 2. GENERALISED

**2.1**    Benign neonatal familial convulsions

Benign neonatal convulsions

Benign myoclonic epilepsy in infancy

Childhood absence epilepsy

Juvenile absence epilepsy

Juvenile myoclonic epilepsy

Epilepsies with grand mal seizures on awakening

Other generalised idiopathic epilepsies

Epilepsies with seizures precipitated by specific modes of activation

Cryptogenic or symptomatic

**2.2**    West syndrome

Lennox-Gastaut syndrome

Epilepsy with myoclonic-astatic seizures

Epilepsy with myoclonic absences

**2.3**    Non-specific etiology

Early myoclonic encephalopathy

Early infantile epileptic encephalopathy with suppression bursts

Other symptomatic generalised epilepsies

**2.4**    Specific syndromes

Epileptic seizures may complicate many disease states

## 3. UNDETERMINED EPILEPSIES

**3.1**    With both generalised and focal seizures

Neonatal seizures

Severe myoclonic epilepsy in infancy

Epilepsy with continuous spike-waves during slow wave sleep

Acquired epileptic aphasia

Other undetermined epilepsies

continued on next page

> **3.2** Without unequivocal generalised or focal features
>
> **4. SPECIAL SYNDROMES**
> **4.1** Situation-related seizures
> Febrile convulsions
> Isolated seizures or isolated status epilepticus
> Seizures occurring only when there is an acute or toxic event
> due to factors such as alcohol, drugs, eclampsia, nonketotic
> hyperglycemia
>
> Epilepsia 1989, 30:389-399

**indication of an abnormal process**

*Epileptic seizures always indicate an abnormal process*, but not all seizures are indicative of a chronic seizure disorder. Under the right circumstances (for example, following a head injury or in the context of acute hypoglycaemia), it may be possible to trigger a seizure in any individual. Acute symptomatic seizures or situation-related seizures, which occur as a result of chemical or physiological insult to the brain, although listed in the ILAE classification of epileptic syndromes (under special syndromes), are not generally considered epileptic disorders in their own right.

## 2.6 What are the characteristics of the main epileptic syndromes?

**age-linked epilepsies**

*Many of the epileptic syndromes start in childhood or adolescence, and are therefore sometimes called age-linked epilepsies.* The more common epileptic syndromes are discussed below.

1.0 Localisation-related epileptic syndromes

1.1 Idiopathic localisation-related syndromes

**Rolandic epilepsy**

*Rolandic epilepsy*, also known as benign partial epilepsy of childhood or centro-temporal epilepsy *is the most common syndrome in this group of seizure disorders*. The onset of seizures is between the ages of 2 and 14 years, usually between 5 and 10 years. This syndrome accounts for about 10-15% of epilepsy in this age group. Children with benign partial epilepsy of childhood usually have simple partial seizures, occasionally with progression to complex partial or secondarily generalised seizures. Seizures tend to occur during the night or on awakening in the morning, and usually involve the face, lips and the tongue.  Consciousness is often preserved. The interictal EEG tracing has a characteristic appearance in this syndrome: it consists of frequent paroxysms of slow spike and wave discharges over the centrotemporal ("rolandic") region, with a normal background rhythm. About 30% of the children have a family history of epilepsy.  There are no neurological or intellectual abnormalities associated with this condition and it has an excellent prognosis for complete seizure remission by the time of puberty.  Long term treatment is usually not required.

*Benign occipital epilepsy is a syndrome with a number of similarities to benign rolandic epilepsy*, but the EEG disturbance is in the occipital lobe and the children may present with visual disturbances during the seizures. **benign occipital epilepsy**

1.2    Symptomatic localisation-related epilepsies and

1.3    Cryptogenic localisation-related epilepsies

*Syndromes in this group are defined by the clinical manifestations of the seizures and by the lobe of the brain in which they originate, regardless of the background aetiology*.  Possible aetiological factors include mesial temporal sclerosis (Ammon's horn), indolent gliomas, cortical dysplasias, cerebral infarction, hamartomas, angiomas, tuberous sclerosis, glial scars and meningiomas.  In about a third of cases no aetiology is found but it is likely that with improvements in imaging techniques, these cryptogenic cases will become progressively less common. **clinical manifestations**

**Temporal lobe seizures**

*Approximately 60-70% of localisation-related epilepsies originate in the temporal lobes*.  Simple partial, complex partial and secondarily generalised *seizures with a large variety of clinical manifestations may occur* as a result of temporal lobe abnormalities.  Because of this diversity they are often very difficult to classify.  The majority of seizures of temporal lobe origin begin in the hippocampus or amygdala.  Autonomic symptoms, impaired consciousness and automatisms are the principal manifestations of these seizures.  Loss of awareness suggests the involvement of both temporal lobes, and may or may not be preceded by a simple partial seizure (an aura). **originate in the temporal lobes**

A strange "rising" sensation in the epigastrium, and anomalies of smell or taste, often of an offensive nature, are common. Patients may undergo autonomic changes, becoming pale or flushed, and with pupillary dilatation, sweating and changes in heart rate. Various psychic phenomena may be experienced by patients having temporal lobe seizures. These include dysmnestic symptoms (for example, déjà vu, jamais vu) and affective experiences (such as exhilaration, fear or anger). Patients may also have auditory or visual hallucinations or illusions. Spontaneous or reactive automatisms may occur, of which oroalimentary (lip-smacking, chewing, swallowing) and motor (drinking, undressing, fumbling, rubbing, and walking) automatisms are the most common. Vocalisation ranging from grunts to repeated words and sentences may also occur. These symptoms may be present in isolation as a simple partial seizure, or in a variety of combinations as complex partial seizures. Both may progress to secondarily generalised seizures.

### Frontal lobe seizures

*About 20-30% of localisation-related epilepsies originate in the frontal lobes.* Simple partial, complex partial and secondarily generalised seizures may occur as a result of frontal lobe discharges. Some frontal lobe seizures, particularly those arising from the motor areas, are easy to classify, while others, particularly those originating from the prefrontal, cingulate and orbitofrontal areas can easily be confused with temporal lobe seizures. Frontal lobe seizures are usually of short duration, often starting and stopping abruptly, and not infrequently occur in clusters.

common manifestations of frontal lobe seizures

*Adversive attacks*, with deviation of the head and eyes to one side at the onset of the attack, *are common manifestations of frontal lobe seizures*. They are often associated with clonic movements of a limb on that side or with limb posturing. Motor automatisms and autonomic symptoms may also occur. Speech arrest may be present, particularly if the seizure originates in the dominant hemisphere, while vocalisation may indicate a non-dominant seizure. Atonic seizures, sometimes causing severe injury, may occur when there is a rapid spread of discharges from one hemisphere to the other. On occasion these evolve into generalised tonic clonic seizures, usually with a rapid recovery afterwards. Post-ictal phenomena such as dysphasia and hemiparesis not infrequently follow seizures of frontal lobe origin: the nature of such phenomena may provide a clue to the location of the epileptic focus.

## Parietal and occipital lobe seizures

*About 10% of all localisation-related epilepsies originate in the parietal and occipital lobes.* Those originating in the parietal lobe often have rather non-specific features, so that the site of origin is not immediately obvious, although somatosensory disturbances may feature in the symptomatology. *Seizures originating in the occipital lobes are characterised by visual phenomena.* These seizures usually present as simple partial seizures but often spread anteriorly leading to complex partial seizures with predominantly frontal or temporal lobe phenomenology. Secondarily generalised convulsions may also occur.

**characterised by visual phenomena**

Somatosensory experiences of parietal origin include localised sensations (tingling, prickling, numbness, crawling or shock-like sensations), pain and changes in temperature. On rare occasions, parietal seizures may manifest themselves as abnormalities of body image, such as a feeling of movement in an immobile limb, a sensation of floating of a body part, or the feeling of absence of a body part. Apraxia, acalculia, alexia, sexual phenomenology and vertiginous sensations may also occasionally occur in parietal lobe epilepsy.

*Elementary visual hallucinations*, especially crude sensations of light and colour, *are the most common manifestations of occipital epilepsy.* These hallucinations may consist of various patterns, usually moving out of the visual field. Transient amaurosis as part of a seizure or as a post-ictal phenomenon may also occur.

**visual hallucinations - manifestations of occipital epilepsy**

## Epilepsia partialis continua

*This is a rare form of severe chronic epilepsy which in the majority of patients starts in the first decade of life.* Patients present with simple partial seizures which become almost continuous: progression to complex partial seizures and secondarily generalised seizures may occur. In some patients, the development of epilepsia partialis continua heralds the onset of a rare condition called Rasmussen's encephalitis (chronic encephalitis and epilepsy). This is an unusual syndrome usually occurring in childhood, and characterised by the development of intractable partial seizures, progressive hemiparesis and intellectual deterioration. Pathologically, changes of chronic encephalitis are seen, almost invariably affecting one cerebral hemisphere only. The aetiology is thought to be viral, although this has never been proven. The condition sometimes

**rare form of severe chronic epilepsy**

seems to stabilise after a period of years, but not before considerable neurological damage has occurred. Other lesions which may cause epilepsia partialis continua at any age include cortical dysplasia, neoplasia, or vascular malformations. Antiepileptic therapy is often ineffective and surgical treatment may be necessary.

2.0    Generalised epilepsies and syndromes

2.1    Idiopathic generalised epilepsy or primary generalised epilepsy

**primary generalised epilepsies**

*The most common of the epileptic syndromes are the generalised idiopathic epilepsies or the primary generalised epilepsies* (2.1 in Table 2). The syndromes contained in this group account for about one third of all epilepsies *and have a typical EEG pattern with paroxysms of generalised "3 per second spike and wave" discharges* (Figure 3) which may be induced by overbreathing and photic stimulation (photosensitivity). Patients often have a family history of generalised epilepsy, suggesting that genetic factors are important. The onset of seizures in this group is usually between the ages of 5 and 15 years, although occasionally they develop in younger children. *Either sex may be affected*.

The seizure types seen in these syndromes are generalised tonic clonic seizures, typical absence seizures and myoclonic seizures, on their own or in different combinations. Within these syndromes, generalised tonic clonic

**tendency for early morning occurrences**

seizures are usually seen much less frequently than myoclonic or absence seizures. *There is a tendency for both generalised tonic clonic convulsions and myoclonic seizures to occur early in the morning*, either on awakening or within half an hour of waking. The majority of patients in this group find that seizures (of any type) may be triggered by sleep deprivation, and in some, photosensitivity is also a feature. Patients who are photosensitive may have seizures in association with flickering lights caused by natural phenomena such as the reflection of the sun on water, travelling in a car along a tree-lined boulevard with the sun in the background, or by artificial causes such as flickering lights in a discotheque, television screens or electronic games. Occasionally a patient's first seizure happens to occur in the context of such a precipitant, which may then be blamed for the development of epilepsy, although underlying photosensitivity can often be demonstrated. It should be stressed, however, that *the majority of people with epilepsy are not photosensitive*, and these people should not be adversely affected by discotheques, computer games, and so on.

Benign neonatal familial convulsions, benign myoclonic epilepsy in infancy and childhood, juvenile typical absence-type epilepsy, juvenile myoclonic epilepsy and epilepsy with generalised tonic clonic convulsions on awakening are all types of generalised idiopathic epilepsy. *The prognosis for full seizure control and long-term remission in all these forms is usually very good as treatment with specific antiepileptic drugs is highly effective.* Most patient may expect to be able to tail off antiepileptic medication after a number of years in remission. *An exception is juvenile myoclonic epilepsy, in which there is a high relapse rate on discontinuation of medication.*

treatment with antiepileptic drugs is highly effective

2.2 and 2.3    Generalised symptomatic or cryptogenic epilepsies

Generalised symptomatic or cryptogenic epilepsies include *the so-called West syndrome and the Lennox-Gastaut syndrome*, which *have some features in common*. Both occur more commonly in males, and have their onset in childhood. In approximately 30% of cases the child is normal until the seizures start, but development then becomes progressively impaired. In the remaining cases, the epileptic condition is preceded by neurological abnormalities or developmental delay. It is believed that a common physiopathologic mechanism is responsible for both conditions, the differences in presentation occurring as a result of the differing degree of brain maturation.

West syndrome and the Lennox-Gastaut syndrome

West syndrome was originally described in 1841 by a physician in his own baby son. *The terms infantile spasms, salaam spasms and hypsarrhythmia have also been used to refer to this syndrome*. The onset is usually around the age of six months (range 3-9 months), and the child may have identifiable brain damage (such as tuberous sclerosis, cortical dysplasia, malformations, or anoxic-ischaemic insults) prior to the onset, but in about one third of cases no aetiology can be found. In this syndrome a characteristic EEG pattern, termed hypsarrhythmia, is seen. This consists of a chaotic pattern of high amplitude irregular slow activity intermixed with multifocal spike and sharp wave discharges. The seizures may be flexor, extensor, or mixed, the latter type being most common. Flexor spasms consist of sudden flexion of the neck, arm and legs. Sudden flexion of the trunk produces so-called "salaam" or "jack-knife" seizures. During extensor spasms, sudden movement of the neck, trunk and legs occurs, while in mixed spasms, there is flexion of the neck, trunk and arms, and extension of the legs. Seizures often occur in clusters,

infantile spasms

particularly soon after the child has been awoken. *The prognosis for West syndrome is poor*. Overall, only about 20% of children make a complete recovery, with death occurring in a further 20% in childhood. Almost two thirds of survivors have ongoing epilepsy, and up to 50% have persistent neurological handicap. The response to treatment with conventional anti-epileptic drugs is poor in West syndrome, but in some children the outcome may be improved if vigabatrin is given early in the condition. This drug appears particularly helpful in children in whom the condition is associated with tuberous sclerosis. Adrenocorticotrophic hormone (ACTH) and nitrazepam may also be helpful in the management of infantile spasms.

**multiple seizure types** *The Lennox-Gastaut syndrome is characterised by multiple seizure types including tonic and atonic seizures and complex absences*. Tonic-clonic convulsions and myoclonic seizures may also occur. It is a rare condition, accounting for perhaps 1% of all new cases of epilepsy, although due to its poor outcome it may represent as many as 10% of cases of severe epilepsy. *Lennox-Gastaut syndrome is frequently associated with* **associated with learning difficulties** *learning difficulties and neuropsychiatric disturbances*. In about half of the cases no definite aetiological factor can be identified, although it is recognised that some of these are symptomatic rather than truly "cryptogenic". A past history of West syndrome is the most common identifiable cause, being present in 30-40% of children. Other causes include brain damage at birth, infections, tumour and severe head trauma. The condition typically has its onset between the ages of 3 and 5 years, though it may start as early as one year or as late as 8 years of age (rarely even older). Patients are at high risk of developing status epilepticus, which may be either tonic-clonic or non-convulsive. *The prognosis of* **poor prognosis** *Lennox-Gastaut syndrome is very poor*, both with regard to seizure control (seizures persisting in 60-80% of patients) and mental development. Cognitive and behavioural problems are very common, and it is unusual for patients ever to lead independent lives.

The EEG pattern in Lennox-Gastaut syndrome is almost invariably abnormal even interictally (Figure 4). The background activity is slow, and 2-2.5Hz spike and wave and polyspike and wave discharges, often most marked over the anterior and posterior head regions, are characteristically seen. Such discharges may sometimes dominate the EEG for hours or days at a time. The complexes are not usually induced by hyperventilation or by photic stimulation. Rhythmic 10Hz spikes are seen particularly during slow-wave sleep.

*The syndrome of epilepsy with myoclonic-astatic seizures has many* *similarities to the Lennox-Gastaut syndrome*, but can be differentiated by the prominence of myoclonic seizures, the fact that the majority of people have a previously normal neurological history, and by the absence of the characteristic EEG pattern. Tonic seizures, characteristic of Lennox-Gastaut syndrome, only occur late in patients in which the condition is severe. In one third of cases there is a family history. The prognosis for mental development and seizure control is rather variable: seizure frequency may provide some indication of the probable overall outcome.

**myoclonic-astatic seizures**

3.0    Epilepsies and syndromes undetermined whether focal or generalised.

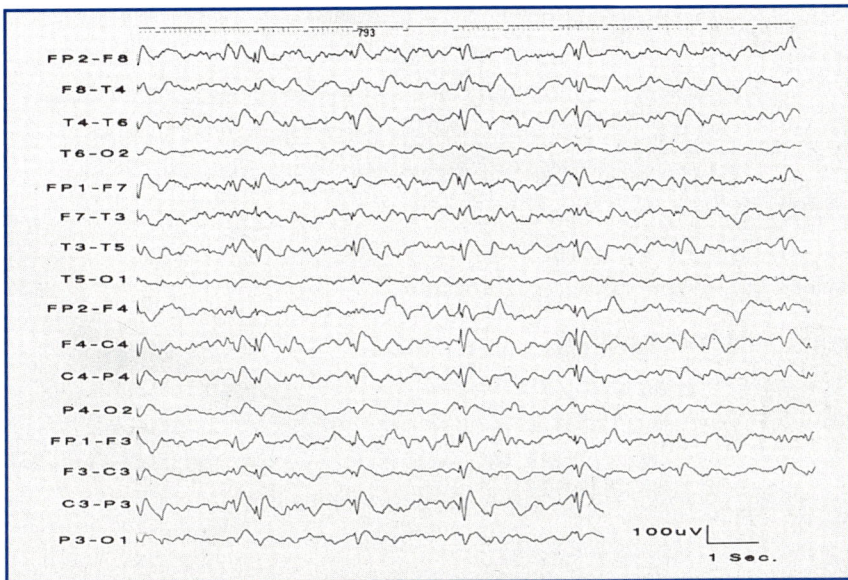

**Figure 4.** *EEG in Lennox-Gastaut syndrome. (Courtesy of Dr Li Li Min).*

## Neonatal seizures

*Neonatal seizures occur in the first 4 weeks of life, in about 0.5% of babies.* The syndrome is defined solely by age of onset, with no regard for the background aetiology or ictal manifestations. Causes of neonatal seizures include infection, anoxia, ischaemia, trauma, metabolic imbalance and nutritional disturbances. In about one quarter of cases no aetiological factor is identified. In a few babies the seizures occur on a genetic basis. Seizures are often subtle and include clonic movements, eye deviation and blinking, usually of short duration: very rarely, more conventional seizure

**first four weeks of life**

immaturity of
the neonatal
brain

types may occur. *The clinical features of the seizures probably reflect the immaturity of the neonatal brain*. The EEG in the neonate is often difficult to interpret, but it may be possible to identify an epileptic focus. The prognosis is related to the underlying pathology, but the overall outcome is not good; approximately 25% die in the first year of life, and about half either carry on having seizures into adult life or have evidence of neurological damage, such as learning disability or cerebral palsy.

25% make a
full recovery

*Only about 25% make a full recovery*. Indicators of poor prognosis include prematurity, early onset of seizures (especially in the first two days of life), focal cerebral lesions or malformations, intracranial bleeding and the presence of a very abnormal EEG. However, two syndromes of "benign" neonatal convulsions have been recognised: benign idiopathic neonatal convulsions ("fifth day fits"), which are said to account for about 5% of neonatal seizures, although some studies have suggested that they may represent one third of all neonatal seizures. Benign familial neonatal convulsions have an autosomal dominant inheritance, the gene being mapped to the long arm of chromosome 20.

**Severe myoclonic epilepsy in infancy**

This is a rare condition which affects infants in the first year of life. It presents with generalised clonic convulsions and myoclonic seizures. The EEG shows generalised spike and wave discharges and marked photosensitivity. Antiepileptic treatment is not effective and the prognosis for seizure control, mental and motor development is poor.

**Acquired epileptic aphasia**

Landau-
Kleffner
syndrome
is a rare
disorder

This condition, also known as *Landau-Kleffner syndrome, is a rare disorder* in which persisting aphasia develops in association with severe focal EEG abnormalities. It occurs more commonly in boys than girls and has its onset in childhood, usually between the ages of four and seven years. The condition usually occurs in children with previously normal development, and the aetiology is unknown. The first sign is usually a progressive acquired aphasia, commonly followed by generalised and partial epileptic seizures, although in about 30% of patients no clinical seizures are noted, while in some children seizures may precede the onset of the language disturbance. Motor speech function is affected, often leading to an almost total mutism. Behaviour disturbances of various types are observed in the majority of patients. The EEG recording shows a multi-focal spike and wave pattern, the epileptic activity most often being seen in the temporal and parieto-occipital regions. *The prognosis for seizure control is usually favourable*, but the outcome of the language disturbance is guarded. In some patients speech may be regained by adulthood, but there may be severe psychosocial consequences as a result of the prolonged aphasia.

## Epilepsy with continuous spike-waves during slow wave sleep

*This condition*, also known as electrical status epilepticus during slow wave sleep (ESES) *is another rare form of childhood epilepsy* which has as its hallmark an EEG pattern consisting of almost continuous slow spike and wave discharges during most of non-REM sleep. The condition usually starts during the first decade of life and the child may present with several different seizure types, both diurnal and nocturnal, including focal motor, complex partial, tonic clonic, absence and atonic seizures. The aetiology is unknown, although about 20-30% of cases are associated with identifiable brain pathology (for example, previous meningitis, birth asphyxia, cytomegalovirus infection). In most patients there is an arrest of mental development at the time of onset, and severe behavioural disturbances may develop. *The prognosis for seizure control is good*, and the electrical status epilepticus generally remits around puberty, although learning difficulties and behavioural disorders usually persist.

4.0    Special syndromes

4.1    Situation-related seizures

Acute head trauma, fever, sleep deprivation, use of convulsant drugs, withdrawal of sedative drugs or alcohol, reversible central nervous system infections, eclampsia, metabolic imbalance, and toxic states can cause epileptic seizures, either single or recurrent, in susceptible individuals, without constituting an epileptic disorder. These seizures are also called acute symptomatic seizures or situation-related seizures. They usually take the form of generalised tonic clonic convulsions. Long-term treatment is not usually required, except in instances in which seizures recur after the triggering factor has been removed or corrected.

**Febrile convulsions**

occur in
febrile illness

*Febrile seizures occur in the context of a febrile illness, often of viral aetiology, in children between the ages of six months and six years.* They affect as many as 3% of children in the general population and there is often a family history of febrile convulsions or epilepsy. The seizures usually take the form of short generalised tonic clonic convulsions, without other features, in toddlers with body temperatures over 38°C, and occur particularly following a rapid rise in temperature. Acute treatment, in addition to supportive management, consists of diazepam, either rectally or intravenously, reducing the child's temperature by means of sponging, cooling with a fan, and paracetamol if necessary, and treatment of the underlying condition if appropriate. Febrile convulsions do not usually require long-term prophylactic treatment unless complications develop. However, parents should be counselled about the risk of recurrences and measures to avoid these. Risks for recurrence include age less than 15 months, epilepsy in first degree relatives, febrile convulsions in first degree relatives, and complex first febrile seizure. In some children intermittent prophylaxis with a benzodiazepine is helpful. EEG is usually not indicated. *The most important differential diagnosis in this condition is with seizures that are triggered by central nervous system infections*

importance
of differential
diagnosis

*such as meningitis, encephalitis and brain abscess.* If there is any doubt about the diagnosis, a lumbar puncture is indicated, provided there are no features to suggest raised intracranial pressure. If there is a suspicion of this, the child should be transferred to a specialist centre with neurosurgical facilities for CT scan before lumbar puncture is performed. In this instance, the need for appropriate antibiotic treatment prior to transfer should be considered.

excellent
prognosis

*In the great majority of children presenting with febrile convulsions, even if recurrent, the overall prognosis is excellent with no further seizures or other problems.* However, in a few children, chronic seizures subsequently develop, so that the risk of epilepsy by the age of 25 years is about 7%. The risk is greatest in children with prolonged convulsions (lasting more than 20-30 minutes), those with previous signs of developmental delay, and those with partial seizures. The probability of epilepsy subsequently developing is also greater in children with a family history of afebrile seizures in a first degree relative.

### 2.7 What factors may precipitate seizures in people with epilepsy?

*In the majority of patients with epileptic seizures, seizures happen in a random fashion and are totally unpredictable.* However, some patients are able to identify certain conditions which may trigger their seizures. If such factors exist and can be identified, measures can be taken to avoid them, thus reducing the likelihood of further attacks. Examples of *factors which may trigger seizures in some patients are flickering lights, sleep deprivation, stressful situations, fear, and anger.* Other people are liable to have seizures when they take certain drugs or alcohol.

**random and totally unpredictable**

**factors which may trigger seizures**

Women with epilepsy often complain that their seizures are more frequent around the time of their menstrual period, probably as a result of hormonal changes and fluid retention. A few of these women are helped by additional medication in the week prior to and during menstruation.

### 2.8 What are nocturnal seizures?

A proportion of people with seizures have most or even all of their attacks during the night. This type of epilepsy may prove difficult to diagnose since seizures are often unwitnessed. *If there is a suspicion of nocturnal seizures, it is important that investigations are carried out since the majority of these patients have seizures of partial origin, and there may be an underlying structural lesion.* There may also be implications for treatment, and many patients with nocturnal seizures without a progressive cause elect not to take antiepileptic drugs.

**seizures of partial origin may have an underlying structural lesion**

### 2.9 What is status epilepticus?

*The great majority of seizures are self-limiting, that is, they stop spontaneously.* On occasion, however, *seizures occur in quick succession, without any period of recovery between one attack and the next, a situation known as status epilepticus.* This may occur with any type of seizure, but it is particularly dangerous if it involves generalised tonic clonic convulsions, when it constitutes a medical emergency.

### 2.10 What are the features of tonic clonic status epilepticus?

*Tonic clonic status epilepticus occurs when a tonic clonic seizure (or recurrent tonic clonic seizures without recovery in between) continues for at least 30 minutes.* The EEG during this period shows almost

**tonic clonic seizures continue for at least 30 minutes**

# EPILEPSY

continuous ictal activity. The annual incidence of tonic clonic status epilepticus has been estimated to be about 20 cases per 100,000 population. Over 60% of cases occur in people with established epilepsy; in the remainder, it occurs as an initial or isolated epileptic phenomenon. *About 5% of all people with epilepsy have at least one episode of tonic clonic status epilepticus in their life.* It is more common in children, in people with learning difficulties and in those with structural cerebral pathology, particularly if this involves the frontal lobes.

**5% have at least one episode of tonic clonic status epilepticus**

In patients with established epilepsy a precipitating factor can be identified in over 50% of cases. *The most important is acute antiepileptic drug withdrawal, either due to poor compliance or under medical supervision.* Other precipitants include withdrawal of other drugs or alcohol, infections, other intercurrent illness or progression of the underlying lesion. In patients presenting with tonic clonic status epilepticus as the first sign of epilepsy, an expanding intracerebral lesion must be ruled out. Other causes of tonic clonic status epilepticus as an initial epileptic phenomenon include head trauma, cerebrovascular disease, and encephalitis.

**the problem of misdiagnosis**

*A common problem in the management of people with tonic clonic status is that of misdiagnosis.* It is our experience that the majority of people referred to tertiary referral centres from other hospitals in presumed status epilepticus do not have the condition. Pseudostatus epilepticus is the most common diagnosis in these patients, and such patients may be identified by EEG monitoring.

Tonic clonic status epilepticus carries a high mortality and neurological morbidity. About 10% of patients with tonic clonic status epilepticus die, usually of the underlying condition. Permanent neurological damage and mental deterioration may result from status, particularly in young children. The longer the duration of the status epilepticus, the more the risk of neurological morbidity is increased.

## 2.11 What are the manifestations of non-convulsive status epilepticus?

**subclinical ictal activity persists for 30 minutes**

*Non-convulsive status epilepticus occurs when prolonged or recurrent minor seizures or subclinical ictal activity persist for 30 minutes or more.* Although any non-convulsive seizure type may cause this form of status, the most common presentations are absence status, atypical absence status and complex partial status. They do not constitute a medical emergency in the same manner as tonic clonic status epilepticus, but it has been argued that prolonged temporal lobe seizure activity may contribute to subsequent memory difficulties. Benzodiazepines are often helpful in treatment, although many cases resolve spontaneously, sometimes with the development of a tonic clonic seizure.

### 2.12 What is absence status?

*Absence status occurs in up to 5% of patients with childhood typical absence-type epilepsy*. The hallmark of absence status is clouding of consciousness and behavioural change which may be present in various degrees of severity. Confusion and disorientation sometimes occur. The eyes may be partially closed, and the patient appears in a trance-like state. *The EEG is diagnostic, showing continuous or almost continuous bilaterally synchronous spike and wave activity, with little or no reactivity to sensory stimuli*. Precipitating features can be identified in a minority of cases, and include withdrawal of medication, hypoglycaemia, hyperventilation, flashing or bright lights, sleep deprivation, fatigue or stress. Most patients have known typical absence epilepsy but occasionally absence status is the first manifestation of epilepsy. Patients may suffer repeated attacks, which in the majority of instances last 12 hours or less, although they may persist for days or weeks. A highly characteristic feature of absence status is the termination of the episode by a generalised tonic clonic seizure. Amnesia is usual for the episode but is variable: it may be punctuated by short patches of recall. The occurrence of episodes of absence status does not seem to prejudice the overall good prognosis of childhood typical absence-type epilepsy.

**continuous bilaterally synchronous spikes**

### 2.13 What are the features of atypical absence status?

Atypical absence status is common amongst patients with the Lennox-Gastaut syndrome. It takes the form of a fluctuating confusional or stuporose state with frequent myoclonic seizures. It is often preceded by alterations in the general physical and psychological state, with changes in the patient's motor activity, mood or intellectual attainment, sometimes lasting for hours or days before the overt status develops, and raising the possibility of subclinical non-convulsive status. The status may evolve gradually, and tonic status may eventually develop. Diffuse slow spike and wave dominates the EEG but is often similar to the usual interictal pattern seen in this condition. The usual therapies for status are generally ineffective. The occurrence of atypical absence status in the Lennox-Gastaut syndrome does not seem to be related to outcome.

### 2.14 How does complex partial status epilepticus present?

*Complex partial status epilepticus* was until recently considered to be a rare form of epilepsy but it is now recognised that episodes of status complicate the course of many partial epilepsies: *they are more common than other types of nonconvulsive status or tonic clonic status*. The clinical features are variable, but the manifestations are not simply prolonged or reiterated versions of isolated complex partial seizures. *The cardinal features of complex partial status are confusion and altered consciousness which may fluctuate or be almost continuous*. The features which may be encountered vary from profound stupor with little response to external stimuli in some patients, to a state in which no discernible confusion is present, but cognitive testing reveals subtle abnormalities. Alterations in posture, convulsive movements, and tonic spasms may all occur intermittently in complex partial status. Adversion of the head and eyes is common. Motor features, including adversion, are more common in frontal status than in temporal complex partial status. Myoclonic jerks, posturing, and orofacial and other motor automatisms also occur. Behavioural changes range from agitation to severe psychomotor retardation and stupor, but in some patients, behaviour may be almost normal. Speech patterns may be markedly altered, with perseveration, confabulation, echolalia, repetitive utterances or stereotyped responses. Patients in a state of complex partial status characteristically say very little, and responses to questions, although eventually appropriate, may show a marked delay between question and answer.

*In some patients, psychotic features are prominent*, with delusions, hallucinations, illogical responses, and often a curious perseverative obsession with opposites, such as black/white, good/bad, left/right. Prolonged dreamy states with altered perception of time or space may occur. *A psychiatric misdiagnosis is common where psychotic features are prominent*, and some patients have histories of psychiatric hospital admissions before the epileptic nature of the event is recognised.

The patient usually has amnesia for the whole episode. Patients with extratemporal status are said to have less alteration of consciousness and amnesia than those with status arising in the temporal lobe.

**confusion and altered consciousness**

**psychotic features are prominent**

**psychiatric misdiagnosis is common**

Complex partial status has no characteristic or consistent scalp EEG pattern. Although seldom normal, the interictal and ictal recordings in complex partial status may be very similar, and a whole range of EEG patterns may be seen. Several different ictal patterns may be demonstrable, including continuous or frequent spike or spike and slow wave discharges, which may be widespread or focal.

# CHAPTER 3

## THE EPIDEMIOLOGY OF EPILEPSY

### 3.1 What are the difficulties of studying the epidemiology of epilepsy?

The epidemiology of epilepsy refers to the characteristics of epilepsy in the community. *There are immense difficulties in establishing precise epidemiological statistics for a heterogeneous condition like epilepsy*. Unlike most ailments, epilepsy is episodic. Between seizures, both the clinical examination and laboratory investigations of patients may be perfectly normal. The diagnosis is, therefore, essentially a clinical one, relying on the patient's account of his seizures, and, often more importantly, on the description given by an eye-witness. The difficulties of diagnosis are compounded by the fact that there is a variety of other conditions in which consciousness may be transiently impaired, which may be confused with epilepsy.

**difficult to establish precise epidemiological statistics**

Another problem in determining the epidemiology of epilepsy lies in the area of case identification. Sometimes patients may be unaware of the nature of their attacks and hence not seek medical help. Patients with infrequent or mild seizures may not receive ongoing medical care and so may be missed in epidemiological surveys. Furthermore, since *in the past there has been a considerable degree of stigma attached to epilepsy*, which to a lesser extent still exists today, patients may be reluctant to admit their condition.

**considerable degree of stigma**

There are few data regarding the incidence and prevalence of specific epileptic syndromes, and most of the rates quoted below relate to the epilepsies in general.

### 3.2 What is the incidence of epilepsy?

*Epilepsy is a very common condition*. Its incidence (the number of new cases per given population per year) has been estimated to be *up to 100 cases per 100,000 persons*, while the cumulative incidence (the risk of having the condition at some time in one's life) is between 2 and 5%.

**up to 100 cases per 100,000 persons**

*No consistent national or racial differences have been found*, although it is thought that the incidence may be higher in developing countries.

The incidence is relatively high in the first two decades of life, but falls over the next few decades, only to increase again in later life, mainly as a result of seizures caused by cerebrovascular disease. The incidence of epilepsy according to age is shown in Figure 5.

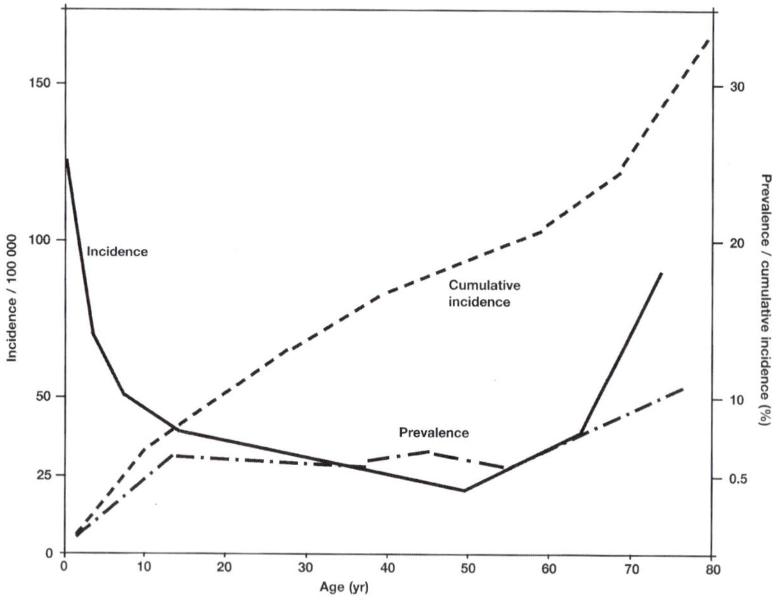

**Figure 5.** *Incidence, prevalence, and cumulative incidence of epilepsy according to age. (Adapted from Hauser WA, Kurland LT. The epidemiology of epilepsy in Rochester, Minnesota, 1935 through 1967. Epilepsia 1975, 16: 1-66).*

### 3.3 What is the prevalence of epilepsy?

The prevalence of epilepsy is the number of cases in the population at a given time. It is important, in defining the prevalence of epilepsy, to distinguish between "active" and "inactive" epilepsy. Epilepsy is usually deemed to be active if the patient has had at least one seizure in recent years (usually the past 2 years, although some investigators consider epilepsy to be active if patients have had seizures within the past 5 years), or if the patient continues to take antiepileptic medication. *Most studies of the prevalence of active epilepsy have estimated the figure to be between 4 and 10 per 1,000* (Figure 5). Cumulative incidence (lifetime prevalence)

**between 4 and 10 per 1,000 persons**

rates are much higher. It is estimated that between 2 and 5% of the population will have a non-febrile seizure at some point in time, and that seizures will recur in over 50%. Almost all reports show higher rates in males than females.

## 3.4 What is the prognosis of epilepsy?

*The prognosis for seizure control is quite good.* As stated above, up to 5% of people will have at least one seizure in their lifetime. The prevalence of active epilepsy is, however, much lower, suggesting that in most patients developing seizures, the condition eventually becomes inactive. *Studies have shown that about 70% to 80% of all people developing epilepsy will eventually become seizure-free and about half will successfully withdraw their medication.* Once a substantial period of remission has been achieved, the risk of further seizures is greatly reduced. A minority of patients (20-30%) will develop chronic epilepsy, and in such cases, treatment is more difficult. Patients with symptomatic epilepsy, more than one seizure type, associated learning difficulties, or neurological or psychiatric disorders are more likely to develop a chronic seizure disorder. 5% of patients with intractable epilepsy will be unable to live in the community or will be dependent on others for their day-to-day needs, often because of associated handicaps. In a minority of patients with severe epilepsy, physical and intellectual deterioration may occur.

## 3.5 What is the risk of recurrence after a first epileptic attack?

The orthodox viewpoint that single seizures should not be equated with epilepsy originates from the findings of early studies of recurrence, which suggested that a considerable proportion of patients with a single seizure had no further attacks. *Reported estimates of the risk of a second attack have varied from 27% by 3 years, to 84% after a variable period of follow-up, depending on how soon the patient is identified after their first seizure and whether treatment is started after the initial event.* Most studies in which patients have been identified very soon after their first attack (within 1 week or so) and not treated indicate that more than 50% of patients will have a recurrence. It is well known that the risk of seizure recurrence is much higher in the first weeks or months after an initial attack. Consequently, if there is a long interval between the first seizure and registration into a recurrence study, a second seizure may have already

occurred and the patient is therefore excluded from the study. From our
own studies, the risk of recurrence also varies depending on the cause of
the seizure (Figure 6) and the length of time for which patients remain
seizure-free after their first attack (Figure 7).

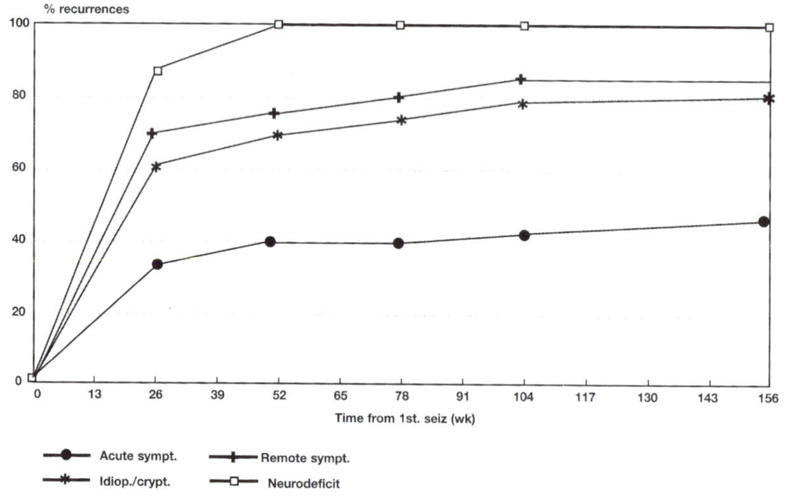

**Figure 6.** *Recurrence after a single seizure according to aetiology. (Adapted from Hart YM, Sander JW, Johnson AL, Shorvon SD. National General Practice Study of Epilepsy: Recurrence after a first seizure. Lancet 1990, 336: 1271-1274).*

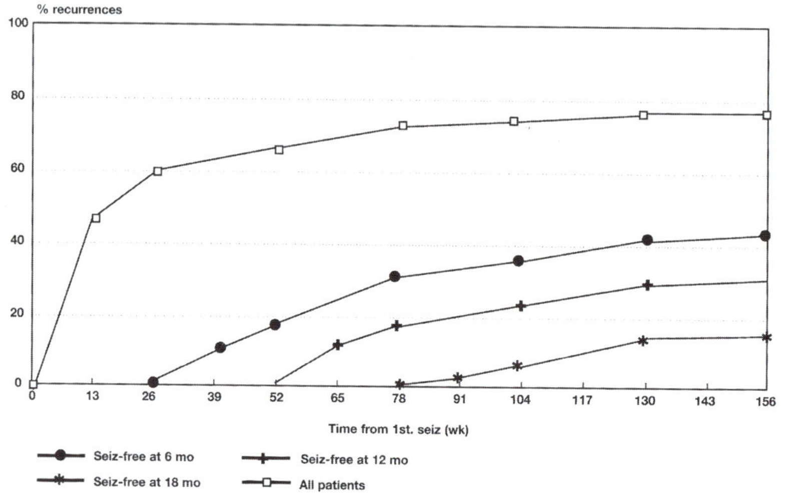

**Figure 7.** *Recurrence after a first seizure according to interval of seizure-freedom from initial event. (Adapted from Hart YM, Sander JW, Johnson AL, Shorvon SD. National General Practice Study of Epilepsy: Recurrence after a first seizure. Lancet 1990, 336: 1271-1274).*

### 3.6 What is the risk of recurrence of seizures after discontinuation of antiepileptic treatment?

*60-70% of patients taking antiepileptic medication will eventually become seizure-free.* Because of the possible long-term side effects of the drugs, it is common clinical practice to consider drug withdrawal after a patient has had a substantial period of remission. Many studies have indicated a risk of relapse in doing so, the probability of this being of the order of 40% in adults and 20% in children after at least two years of freedom from seizures.

### 3.7 What is the mortality of epilepsy?

Epilepsy is often assumed to be a benign condition with a low mortality. Although this is usually the case, *it does carry an increased mortality*, particularly in the case of younger patients and those with severe epilepsy.

**increased mortality in younger patients**

### 3.8 Who is at risk of death from epilepsy?

It has consistently been reported that mortality rates are higher for males than females, although so far no convincing explanation has been advanced for this. The greatest increase in mortality rate is in those people aged less than 40 years, a group which has the smallest mortality in the general population. Conversely, the group in which epilepsy increases the risk of death least is among people aged 75 years or more, those people with the highest mortality rate from other causes.

*The overall mortality rate has been estimated at two to three times greater than that of the general population*, the increased risk being largely limited to the first 10 years after diagnosis. This suggests that the increased mortality is in part due to the underlying cause of epilepsy (brain tumours, head injury, vascular events, and so on), and this view is reinforced by the fact that even patients in whom seizures are completely controlled have an increased risk of death. Nonetheless, idiopathic generalised convulsions also confer an increased mortality.

**mortality rate greater than in the general population**

*Seizure type seems also to be relevant*. The mortality of patients whose only seizure type is absence seizures is little different from that of the general population, while in patients with myoclonic seizures mortality is increased four-fold. Higher mortality rates for non-whites of either sex,

**seizure type is relevant**

both for deaths due to and related to epilepsy, have been reported in the USA. This may, however, be related to socio-economic factors; infant mortality rates, a well-accepted measure of socio-economic deprivation, are almost twice as high amongst Afro-Americans as in the white population.

### 3.9 What are the causes of death in epilepsy?

**common causes of death**

*Common causes of death in people with epilepsy include chest infections, neoplasia, and deaths directly related to seizures.* Bronchopneumonia is an important cause of death of patients with epilepsy, particularly among the elderly although it is by no means confined to this age group. It seems likely that its occurrence in younger people is related to aspiration during a seizure, although this hypothesis has not been formally tested. Deaths from cancer in people with epilepsy have been shown to be increased in several studies. Idiosyncratic side effects of some antiepileptic drugs have been associated with the death of patients, but are extremely rare events. Deaths directly related to seizures fall into several categories: status epilepticus, seizure-related death, sudden unexpected death and accidents. There is an extensive literature on death in status epilepticus, which is estimated to occur in about 10% of all cases of generalised tonic clonic status. Death due to seizures is often given as an explanation used when the patient dies during or shortly after a seizure, when there is no evidence for status epilepticus and when after autopsy no other explanation can be found. An arbitrary distinction is usually made between these patients and those dying from "sudden unexpected death".

**unexpected death for which no cause is found**

*Sudden unexpected death in epilepsy is defined as a non-traumatic unwitnessed death occurring in a patient with epilepsy who had been previously relatively healthy, for which no cause is found even after a thorough post-mortem examination.* The occurrence of sudden unexpected death in epilepsy has long been recognised, being reported before the introduction of modern antiepileptic drugs. Suggested explanations for the cause of death have included suffocation during a seizure, deleterious action of antiepileptic drugs, autonomic seizures affecting the heart, and the release of endogenous opioids, although the pathophysiology (if indeed there is a single mechanism) is still unknown. *The annual mortality rate of sudden death has been variably estimated at one in two hundred to one in twelve hundred people with epilepsy.* The rate may be even higher among people aged 20 to 40 years, and higher still if only patients with uncontrolled seizures are selected.

*Another possible cause of mortality and morbidity in people with epilepsy is as a result of accidents during seizures* or as a consequence of a seizure. The precise extent of this problem is unknown. However, mortality rates for traumatic death have been shown to be increased, indicating that accidents and trauma are a more frequent cause of death in patients with epilepsy than in the general population. There is also an increased mortality from drowning among people with epilepsy. This may occur either in the bath or while swimming. It has been suggested that the rate may be higher in countries where bathing is favoured over showering, although this has never been properly investigated.

**accidents during seizures**

*Mortality rates also indicate that patients with epilepsy are at a higher risk of committing suicide than the general population.* Patients with temporal lobe epilepsy and severe epilepsy, or epilepsy with a handicap have a much greater risk of suicide, 25 times in the cases of temporal lobe epilepsy and five times for severe epilepsy. There seems to be some evidence that risk may decline with duration of the condition.

**higher risk of suicide**

### References

Sander JW. Some aspects of prognosis in the epilepsies.
Epilepia 1993; 34:1007-1016.

Sander JW, Shorvon SD. The epidemiology of the epilepsies.
Journal of Neurology, Neurosurgery and Psychiatry 1996; 61:433-443.

Nashef L, Sander JW, Shorvon SD. The mortality of epilepsy.
In: Pedley TA, Meldrum BS, (eds.). Recent Advances in Epilepsy. Vol 6.,
Edinburgh: Churchill Livingstone, 1995: 271-87.

# CHAPTER 4
## THE AETIOLOGY OF EPILEPSY

### 4.1 What is an "epileptic threshold"?

*Epileptic seizures are produced by abnormal discharges of neurons, and may be a manifestation of many different conditions which modify neuronal function or which cause pathological changes in the brain.* A plethora of environmental, genetic, pathological and physiological factors may be involved in the development of seizures. The genetic effect on susceptibility to seizures (seizure threshold) is likely to be multifactorial, and may also vary according to the stage of brain maturation. This "seizure threshold" probably determines the strength of stimulus required to generate an epileptic seizure.

*factors involved in the development of seizures*

*A number of precipitants for epileptic seizures are recognised.* These may trigger seizures in patients with established epilepsy, and occasionally in susceptible individuals who have not had previous seizures. Among these precipitants are alcohol withdrawal, fever, head injury, infections, metabolic disturbances, photosensitivity, sleep deprivation, stress and the use of certain drugs. A variety of static or progressive pathological changes, either congenital or acquired, may predispose to seizures. In addition, a number of inherited conditions, which seem to be neurochemically determined, may express themselves solely through epileptic seizures. *It is likely that the dynamic interaction between the seizure threshold and seizure precipitants will determine an individual's propensity to have situation-related epileptic seizures*, which may be isolated or recurrent, *and also to develop a chronic epileptic disorder*.

*interaction between seizure threshold and precipitants*

### 4.2 What are the most common aetiologies of epilepsy?

*The probable aetiology depends on the age of the patient and the type of seizures.* The most common acquired causes in young infants are hypoxia or birth asphyxia, perinatal intracranial trauma, metabolic disturbances, congenital malformations of the brain, and infection. In young children and adolescents, idiopathic or primary epilepsies account for the majority of seizure disorders, although trauma and infection also

*aetiology depends on age and type of seizures*

play a role. *Febrile seizures*, which are usually short, generalised tonic clonic convulsions occurring during the early phase of a febrile disease, *are common in children aged between six months and five years,* and *need to be distinguished from seizures triggered by central nervous system infections causing fever*, such as meningitis and encephalitis. Unless febrile seizures are prolonged, focal, recurrent, or there is a background of neurological handicap, *the prognosis is excellent*, and it is unlikely that the child will develop chronic epilepsy.

**causes of adult onset epilepsy**

*The causes of adult onset epilepsy are very wide.* Both idiopathic epilepsy and epilepsy due to birth trauma may also begin in early adulthood. Other important causes of seizures in adulthood are head injury, alcohol abuse, brain tumours and cerebrovascular disease. In developing countries, parasitic disorders such as cysticercosis and malaria may also be important causal agents for epilepsy. Brain tumours are responsible for the development of epilepsy in up to one third of patients between the ages of 30 and 50 years. Over the age of 50, cerebrovascular disease is the most common cause of epilepsy and may be present in up to half of the patients.

### 4.3 What are the most common genetically determined epilepsies?

**idiopathic generalised or primary generalised group of conditions**

*The idiopathic generalised or primary generalised group of conditions are probably the most common of the genetically determined epilepsies.* The precise mode of inheritance for most of these conditions is unknown at this stage although an autosomal dominant trait is thought to be responsible in some cases. Genetic mapping has shown the gene for juvenile myoclonic epilepsy to lie on chromosome 6, while that for benign neonatal convulsions lies on chromosome 20. It is likely that the mode of inheritance of other conditions in this group will soon be clarified.

Other inherited epileptic conditions which present with seizures as the sole clinical manifestation including the idiopathic localisation-related epilepsies (such as benign rolandic epilepsy) are also thought to be inherited in an autosomal dominant mode with incomplete penetrance.

In addition to these inherited conditions which have seizures as their main clinical expression, there is a large number of inherited disorders, most of them rare, which present as neurological or systemic illnesses of which epileptic seizures form a part. The most common of these disorders are two neurocutaneous conditions (phakomatoses): tuberous sclerosis and neurofibromatosis. Down's syndrome (trisomy 21) is also not infrequently accompanied by seizures, particularly in later life. The progressive myoclonic epilepsies are a group of disorders characterised by the development of myoclonic and sometimes other seizures in association with other clinical manifestations which may include ataxia and progressive dementia. Rare inherited degenerative brain disorders and inborn errors of metabolism such as adrenoleukodystrophy, Alpers' disease and Tay-Sachs disease, phenylketonuria, porphyria and neuronal ceroid-lipofuscinosis may also cause seizures.

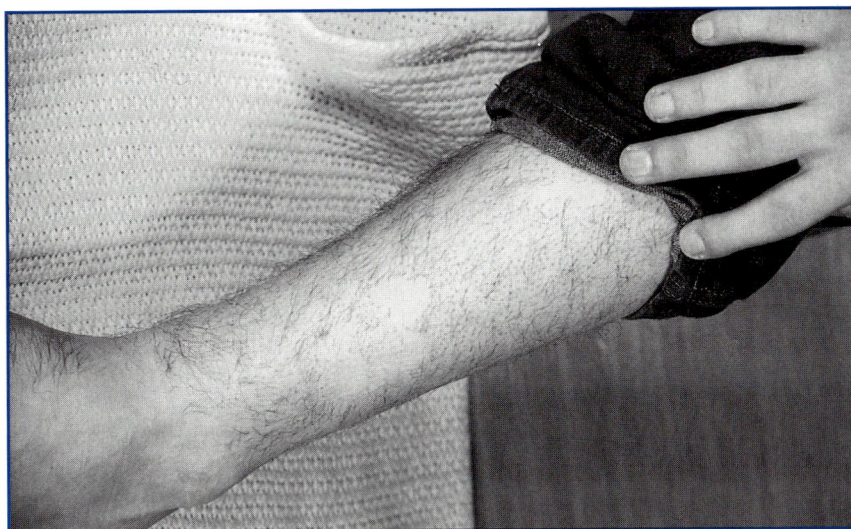

**Figure 8.** *Hypomelanotic patch seen in tuberous sclerosis.(Courtesy of Professor SD Shorvon).*

### 4.4 What is tuberous sclerosis?

*Tuberous sclerosis* (sometimes also known as adenoma sebaceum, epiloia, or Bourneville's Disease) *is inherited as an autosomal dominant condition. Linkage studies have suggested loci on chromosomes 9 and 11.* Manifestations of the disease include partial seizures, cutaneous lesions (including facial angiofibromas, periungual fibromas, fibrous plaques of the scalp, shagreen patches and hypomelanotic areas (Figure 8) and learning difficulties in varying degrees of severity depending on the penetrance of the gene. The most severe forms usually start in early childhood, sometimes presenting as West syndrome. In such cases severe learning difficulties are the rule. At the less severe end of the spectrum,

**inherited as an autosomal dominant condition**

patients may be of average intelligence with very few signs of the disease. Seizures affect more than 90% of patients and on occasion are the only clinical manifestation. The characteristic lesions seen on neuroimaging are subependymal nodules consisting of glial tissues which may be calcified ("tubers"). These are usually most prominent in the temporal lobes and are commonly situated adjacent to the ventricles. Prognosis for complete seizure control is usually guarded.

### 4.5 What are the features of neurofibromatosis?

autosomal
dominant
disease

*Neurofibromatosis (von Recklinghausen's disease) is an autosomal dominant disease* in which spots of skin hyperpigmentation (café au lait patches) are combined with multiple neurofibromas arising from Schwann cells. There is a wide spectrum of severity. Mild cases may be asymptomatic, while at the other end of the spectrum major skin deformities and florid neurological manifestations are seen. Partial epileptic seizures occur in less than 10% of cases and are usually due to brain tumours such as meningioma, glioma or neurinoma, which are found in patients with neurofibromatosis at a much higher frequency than in the general population.

**Table 3.** *Some causes of progressive myoclonus epilepsy.*

Unverricht-Lundborg disease
Lafora body disease
Neuronal ceroid lipofuscinosis
Sialidoses
Myoclonus epilepsy with ragged red fibres (MERRF)

### 4.6 What are the progressive myoclonic epilepsies?

Lafora's
disease and
familial Baltic
myoclonus

This is a heterogeneous group (Table 3) comprising several degenerative diseases which have in common the occurrence of myoclonic seizures, generalised tonic clonic convulsions and progressive intellectual deterioration, although the latter may be mild in some of the conditions. *Lafora's disease and familial Baltic myoclonus are the most common disorders* in this group and both have a guarded prognosis for the control of the myoclonus and also for long-term survival. The generalised tonic clonic convulsions, however, are readily treatable with antiepileptic drugs.

Mitochondrial myopathies, particularly the MERFF (Myoclonic Epilepsy and Ragged Red Fibres) and the MELAS (Myoclonic Epilepsy, Lactic Acidosis and Stroke) syndromes are also associated with progressive myoclonic epilepsy: both have a guarded prognosis.

## 4.7 What are the most common symptomatic or acquired epilepsies?

*Common causes of symptomatic epilepsies include head trauma, birth trauma, cerebrovascular disorders, brain neoplasms, anoxia, craniotomy, brain infections including acquired immune deficiency syndrome, and some degenerative brain diseases*. In developing countries, parasitic infestations such as malaria, neurocysticercosis and paragonimiasis are important causes of acquired epilepsy. It is probable that cortical dysgenesis and hippocampal sclerosis, which have been increasingly associated with chronic epilepsy, are also acquired lesions. Most epilepsies starting in adult life are symptomatic and investigations to detect the underlying aetiology are mandatory.

**common causes of acquired epilepsies**

## 4.8 What is the role of head injury in the development of symptomatic epilepsy?

Head trauma is an important cause of symptomatic partial seizures. Post-traumatic epilepsy accounts for up to 10% of all cases of epilepsy in some series. *The likelihood of developing epilepsy after head trauma depends on the severity of the injury and the presence of complicating factors, including prolonged loss of consciousness, post-traumatic amnesia of more than 30 minutes, intracranial bleeding, penetration of a missile, or a depressed skull fracture*. It is very unusual for seizures to develop unless one of these factors is present. It is thought that deposits of haemosiderin due to local bleeding may be responsible for the development of an epileptic focus at the site of injury. In the majority of cases seizures start within two years of the injury. The response to treatment is variable. Seizures occurring immediately after the injury or within the first week do not usually presage the development of chronic epilepsy.

**severity of the injury and the presence of complicating factors**

*Prophylactic antiepileptic drug treatment after head injury has often been advocated* in an attempt to prevent the subsequent development of epilepsy. There is, *however,* no clear evidence that it is effective, and *most authorities now start treatment only if seizures occur.*

### 4.9 What is the role of birth trauma in the development of symptomatic epilepsy?

**direct trauma or anoxia** *Brain injury occurring during labour may cause symptomatic epilepsy, either as a result of direct trauma, or because of anoxia.* The outcome is variable and to a large extent dependent on the severity of the injury. Birth injury was a common cause of epilepsy in the past, but with improvements in antenatal care and midwifery over the past few decades, this is no longer the case. The seizures are partial in nature, the epileptic focus being at the site of injury. Anoxia often causes more extensive brain damage and the seizures may be generalised.

### 4.10 What is the role of cerebrovascular disease in the development of symptomatic epilepsy?

**thromboem- bolic events and cerebral haemorrhage** *Thromboembolic events and cerebral haemorrhage are important causes of symptomatic epilepsy starting in later life*: they are responsible for as many as 50% of cases in this age-group. Seizures are almost always partial, and usually start within a year of the cerebrovascular event although sometimes they may precede the stroke, suggesting previous silent ischaemic episodes. Seizures occurring during or immediately after a stroke are not predictive of the late development of epilepsy. It has been estimated that *approximately 15% of people with strokes will* eventually *develop epileptic seizures, which are usually controlled with antiepileptic drugs*.

Vascular malformations and cerebral aneurysms may also cause symptomatic epilepsy, whether or not haemorrhage has occurred. Acute subarachnoid haemorrhage may also lead to situation-related (acute symptomatic) seizures.

Sturge-Weber syndrome (encephalotrigeminal syndrome) is characterised by the presence of capillary or cavernous haemangiomas within the cutaneous distribution of the trigeminal nerve, with venous haemangiomas in the parietal, occipital and frontal regions on the same side. Either the cutaneous manifestations or the intracranial lesions may occur independently. Sturge-Weber syndrome is often associated with severe partial seizures, and the prospect for full seizure control is poor. Other neurological manifestations may also be present.

### 4.11 What is the role of brain tumours in the genesis of symptomatic epilepsy?

*Intracranial tumours, whether benign or malignant, may cause epileptic seizures.* Such tumours may arise in the brain or meninges (usually gliomas or meningiomas) or may be metastatic from a distant site. Intracranial neoplasms are responsible for about 20% of seizures starting between the ages of 30 and 50 years, and about 10% of seizures starting after the age of 50 years. The seizures are always partial in nature and are due either to mass effect or damage to surrounding cortical tissues. *The likelihood of a tumour causing seizures seems to be related to its histological type and the location.* The prognosis is largely dependent on the nature and site of the tumour.

**intracranial tumours may cause epileptic seizures**

Hamartomas, which have been classified as brain tumours by some, are occasionally found in tissue resected from patients undergoing surgery for temporal lobe epilepsy. They consist of abnormal masses of intertwined neuronal, vascular and glial tissues and are probably developmental anomalies lacking neoplastic characteristics.

### 4.12 Do infections of the brain cause chronic epilepsy?

*Any intracranial infection, whether viral, bacterial or fungal, can cause seizures which may continue after the infection has been successfully treated.* Pre- and peri-natal infections may be implicated in addition to post-natal encephalitis or meningitis. The seizures are partial, the epileptic foci occurring as a result of localised pathological changes. The severity of the epileptic disorder usually depends on the nature of the infection and the extent of the damage.

**viral, bacterial or fungal infection may cause seizures**

*Meningitis is the most common intracranial infection.* It is common in young children but also affects adolescents and older age groups. Epilepsy is an unusual complication of acute bacterial meningitis, occurring mainly in people given inadequate or late treatment. *Seizures are usually partial,* and the prognosis for total seizure control is in most cases guarded.

**meningitis**

*Intracranial tuberculosis* can cause cortical and meningeal tuberculomas which may present *with seizures sometimes developing only years after the primary infection.* The response to medical treatment is usually poor and surgery should be considered in selected cases.

**fungal infections** *Fungal infections of the central nervous system are a very rare cause of epilepsy*, the most common being cryptococcosis and blastomycosis. *Cryptococcosis occurs in patients with such underlying conditions as diabetes, sarcoidosis, lymphomas and acquired immune deficiency syndrome (AIDS)*, in more than 50% of cases. Blastomycosis, which affects males more than females, is prevalent in tropical and sub-tropical regions including the southeast of the United States. It should be suspected in any patient who has visited Africa or Central or South America and develops seizures in the context of an ill-defined systemic illness.

**viral encephalitis** *Viral encephalitis, especially due to herpes, may cause epileptic seizures* both during the acute phase and as a late complication. During the acute phase generalised tonic-clonic seizures are common, often resulting in status epilepticus. Seizures developing after an encephalitic process are usually partial and are often intractable to medical treatment.

Intrauterine and perinatal infections caused by such agents such as toxoplasmosis, rubella and syphilis may cause extensive cortical damage, and severe partial epilepsy may result if the child survives.

A rare chronic unilateral encephalitic process known as Rasmussen's syndrome (chronic encephalitis and epilepsy) is characterised by the development of partial seizures and frequently epilepsia partialis continua, progressive hemiparesis and intellectual deterioration. Possible aetiologies include a viral infection, or an autoimmune process.

Brain abscesses are rare, and are often fatal. Partial epileptic seizures develop in about three quarters of survivors, and are usually very severe and intractable, particularly with lesions located in the frontal and temporal lobes.

### 4.13 In what circumstances do seizures occur in acquired immune deficiency syndrome?

**HIV testing should be considered in patients with risk factors** *Involvement of the central nervous system eventually occurs in the majority of people developing AIDS.* It may take the form of opportunistic infection or neoplastic lesions. An encephalopathy which seems to be caused by the human immunodeficiency virus (HIV) itself has also been recognised. Any of these conditions may present with epileptic seizures, either as the initial manifestation or late in the disease. Seizures due to opportunistic infections and neoplasms are usually of a partial nature, while those due to HIV encephalopathy are usually generalised tonic- clonic convulsions. The diagnosis, particularly when a seizure is the first manifestation, may be difficult, and *HIV testing should be considered in patients with risk factors*.

## 4.14 Which parasitic infections may be associated with epilepsy?

*Epilepsy may occur in the course of a number of parasitic disorders,* including neurocysticercosis (due to Taenia solium), malaria (Plasmodium falciparum), schistosomiasis (Schistosoma japonicum), paragonimiasis or endemic haemoptysis (Paragonimus westermani), toxocariasis (Toxocara canis), onchocerciasis or river blindness (Onchocerca volvulus) and American trypanosomiasis or Chagas' disease (Trypanosoma cruzi). *Such infections may be responsible for the high incidence of epilepsy in some parts of the tropical world.* The most common to be associated with epilepsy are neurocysticercosis and falciparum malaria.

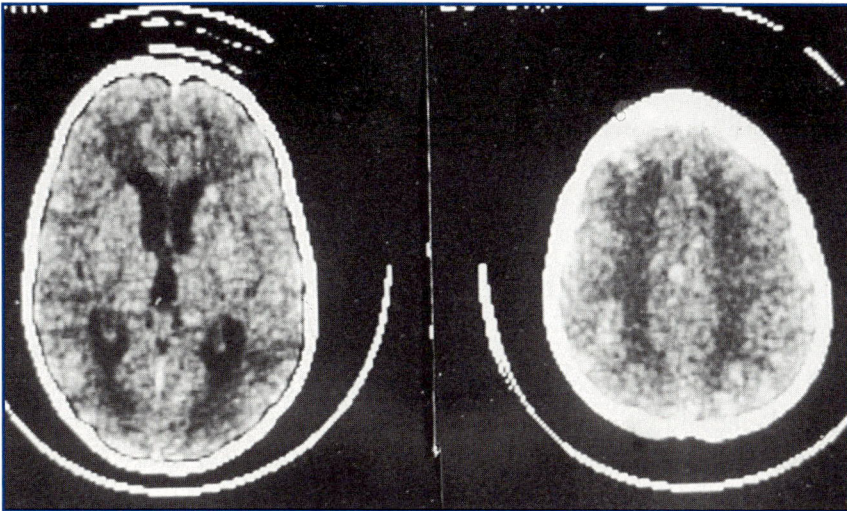

**Figure 9.** *CT scan showing infection with cysticercosis. (Courtesy of Dr Paulo Bittencourt).*

Neurocysticercosis is the most common acquired cause of epilepsy in some developing countries, particularly in Latin America. This occurs when man becomes the intermediate host for Taenia solium (the pork tapeworm) through the ingestion of eggs contained in human faeces. Cysts containing an embryo may emerge in any area of the cerebrum, ventricles or subarachnoid space of the infested patient (Figure 9), leading to a variety of neurological signs including partial seizures, which may sometimes be the only manifestation. Prognosis is variable and usually depends on the number and location of the cysts. Neurocysticercosis should be suspected in any individual developing partial seizures who has lived in or visited an endemic area.

*Cerebral malaria, which is the most important complication of falciparum malaria, may first present as status epilepticus*. It carries a high mortality and morbidity. Survivors often have partial seizures which respond poorly to treatment with antiepileptic drugs.

### 4.15 What is the risk of epilepsy after craniotomy?

**neurosurgical procedures are associated in about 10% of cases**

*Neurosurgical procedures involving the supratentorial region are associated with the development of epileptic seizures in about 10% of cases*. The incidence, however, varies depending on the location and the condition for which the craniotomy was performed. In patients with uncomplicated aneurysm surgery it may be as low as 5%, while it can be as high as 90% following surgery for cerebral abscess. The seizures are usually partial, and occur within the first year in the majority of cases. Prophylactic antiepileptic drug treatment after craniotomy has been advocated although there is no evidence that it reduces the risk of developing epilepsy.

### 4.16 Can epilepsy occur in degenerative brain diseases?

Epilepsy may sometimes complicate degenerative brain conditions such as Alzheimer's disease, Huntington's chorea, striatonigral degeneration and Jakob-Creutzfeld disease. Patients with Alzheimer's disease are at considerably increased risk of developing epileptic seizures, with as many as 20% of patients being affected.

### 4.17 What proportion of patients with multiple sclerosis develop seizures?

**4% of people with multiple sclerosis develop epileptic seizures**

*Epileptic seizures occur in about 4% of people with multiple sclerosis and are rarely the first manifestation of the condition*. Seizures are usually partial in nature although generalised tonic clonic convulsions may also occur. *The prognosis for seizure control is usually good* although the overall prognosis is that of the background condition, that is, highly varied and unpredictable.

## 4.18 What is the risk of epilepsy following vaccination?

*An allergic reaction to vaccine components very occasionally leads to an acute encephalopathy* which may cause acute symptomatic seizures and also result in chronic epilepsy. Such a reaction has been reported following vaccination against rabies, smallpox and whooping-cough (pertussis). *It is however, extremely rare, and is becoming even more uncommon as more purified and less antigenic vaccines are used.*

**allergic reaction may lead to acute encephalopathy**

It is important to note that *the incidence of epilepsy is at its highest in early childhood*, the age at which most vaccinations are carried out, *and* therefore *some children will develop seizures in temporal association with vaccination by coincidence*. Other children experience a febrile reaction to some vaccinations and may have a febrile seizure as a result, without long-term sequelae.

The presence of a history of epileptic seizures or of a family history of epilepsy in a child is no longer considered a contraindication to immunisation, since the risk of the condition for which the inoculation is being given is greater than that of vaccination.

## 4.19 Under what circumstances does anoxia cause epilepsy?

Anoxia sufficiently severe to cause epilepsy is probably most common in the perinatal period. It is usually associated with severe morbidity, with epileptic seizures being a common manifestation. Anoxia may also occur in the course of a cardiac or respiratory arrest, and may be followed by the development of chronic myoclonic seizures.

## 4.20 What are cortical dysplasias?

*Errors in neuronal migration during embryogenesis may result in cortical dyplasias or dysgenesis*: in an analogy with the skin these would constitute the "bumps and blemishes" of the brain. Cortical dysgenesis was until recently considered to be rare: however, with the development of modern neuroimaging techniques, particularly high resolution magnetic resonance scanning, it is being recognised with increasing frequency. Cortical dysplasias can be divided into four broad categories: gyral abnormalities, heterotopias, focal cortical dysplasias including microdysgenesis, and proliferative dysgenesis.

**errors in neuronal migration during embryogenesis**

Gyral abnormalities include agyria or lissencephaly (absence of gyri over the whole brain), schizencephaly (Figure 10, with 3-D reconstruction, Figure 11) (in which clefts extend from the cortex to the ventricular surface) and localised areas of macrogyria (Figure 12) or polymicrogyria (Figure 13). Heterotopias consist of bands or nodules of normal neurons which are located incorrectly, usually subcortically (Figures 14, 15). Focal cortical dysplasias and microdysgenesis are characterised by clusters of abnormal neurons usually positioned in aberrant locations (Figure 16). Among the proliferative dysgeneses are dysembryoplastic neuroepithelial tumours (Figure 17). These are benign congenital lesions which are easily confused with low-grade gliomas. They are predominantly cortical, often multinodular, may contain cystic components and have associated areas of cortical dysgenesis.

**aetiology of cortical dysplasias is unknown**

*The aetiology of cortical dysplasias is unknown at this stage*, but potential causes are thought to include intrauterine infection, maternal illness or exposure to toxins at 8-16 weeks of gestation when neuronal migration occurs, or insults occurring in the last trimester of gestation when gyral formation takes place.

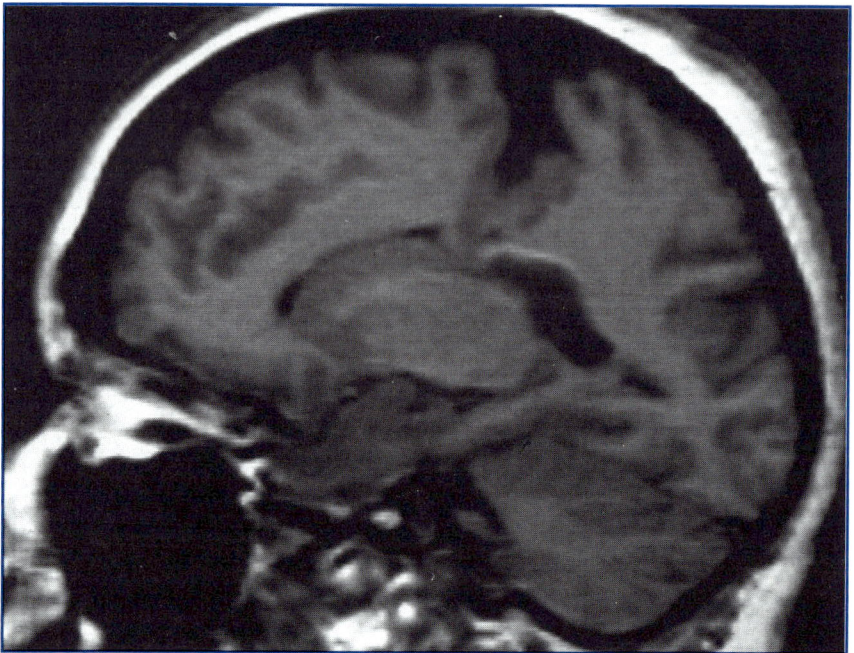

**Figure 10.** *MRI scan showing schizencephaly. (Courtesy of Dr Raymond Ali).*

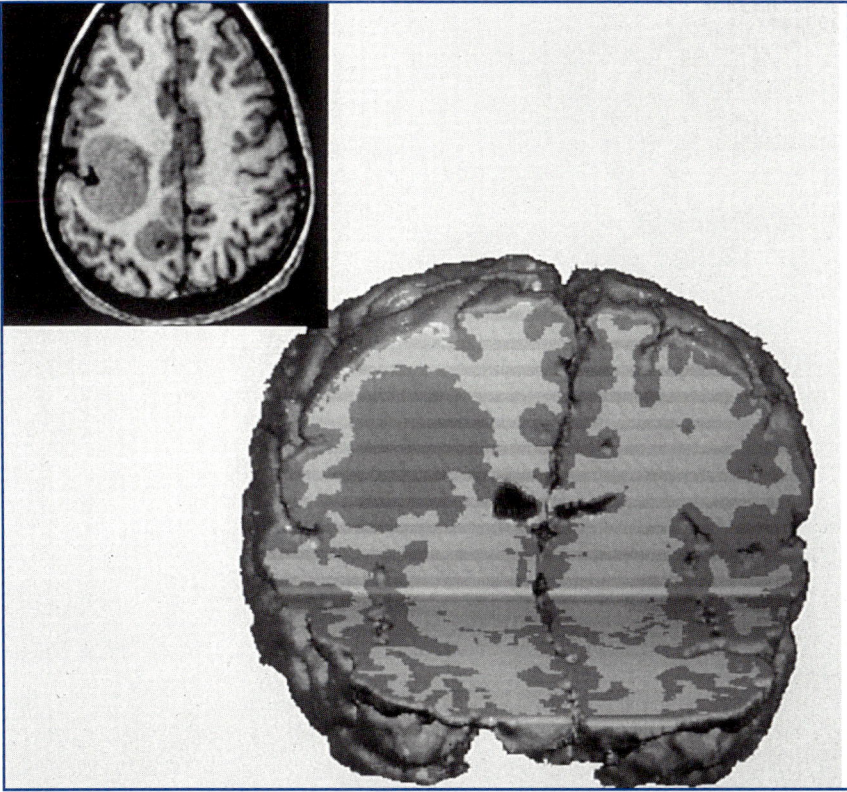

**Figure 11.** *MRI scan showing schizencephaly with 3-D reconstruction. (Courtesy of Dr Sanjay Sisodiya).*

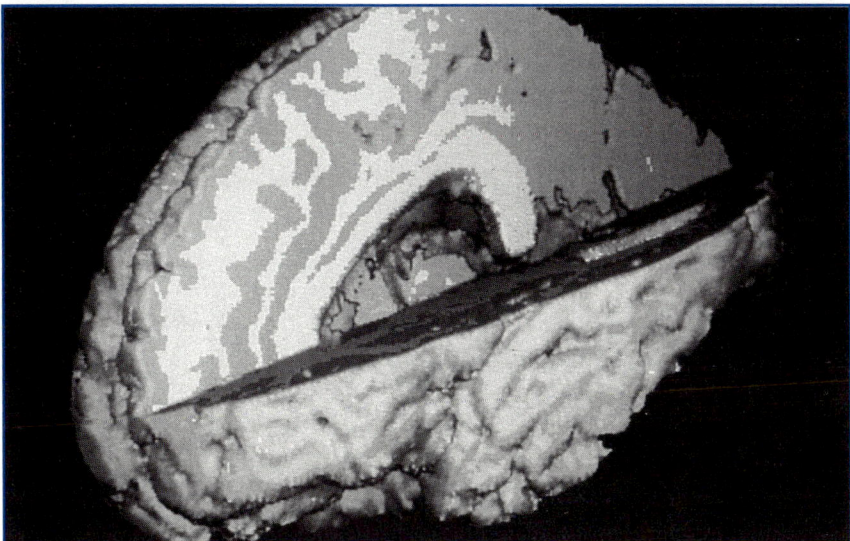

**Figure 12.** *MRI scan showing macrogyria. (Courtesy of Dr Sanjay Sisodiya).*

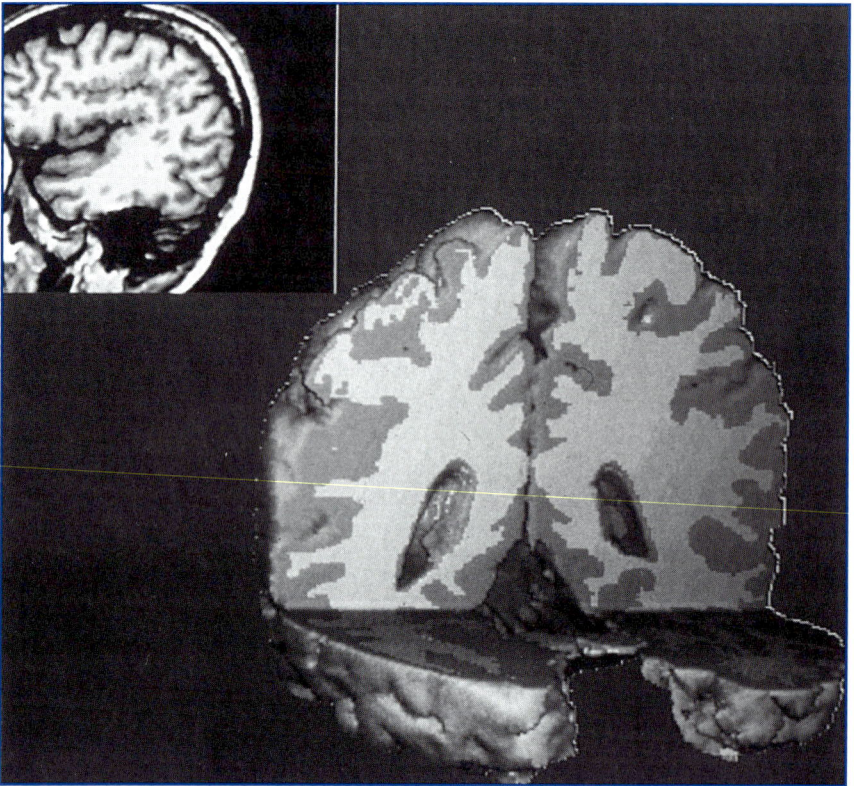

**Figure 13.** *MRI scan showing polymicrogyria. (Courtesy of Dr Sanjay Sisodiya).*

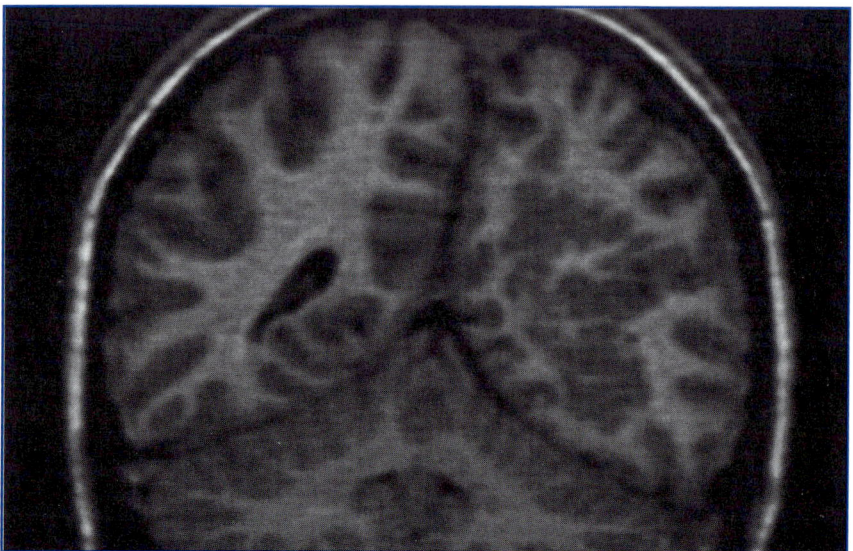

**Figure 14.** *MRI scan showing occipitotemporal heterotopia. (Courtesy of Dr Sanjay Sisodiya).*

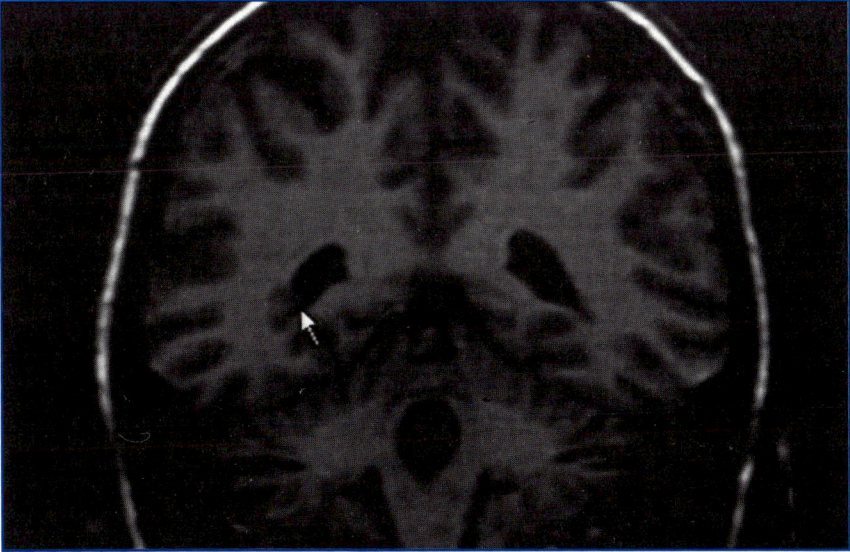

**Figure 15.** *MRI scan showing nodular subependymal heterotopia. (Courtesy of Dr Raymond Ali).*

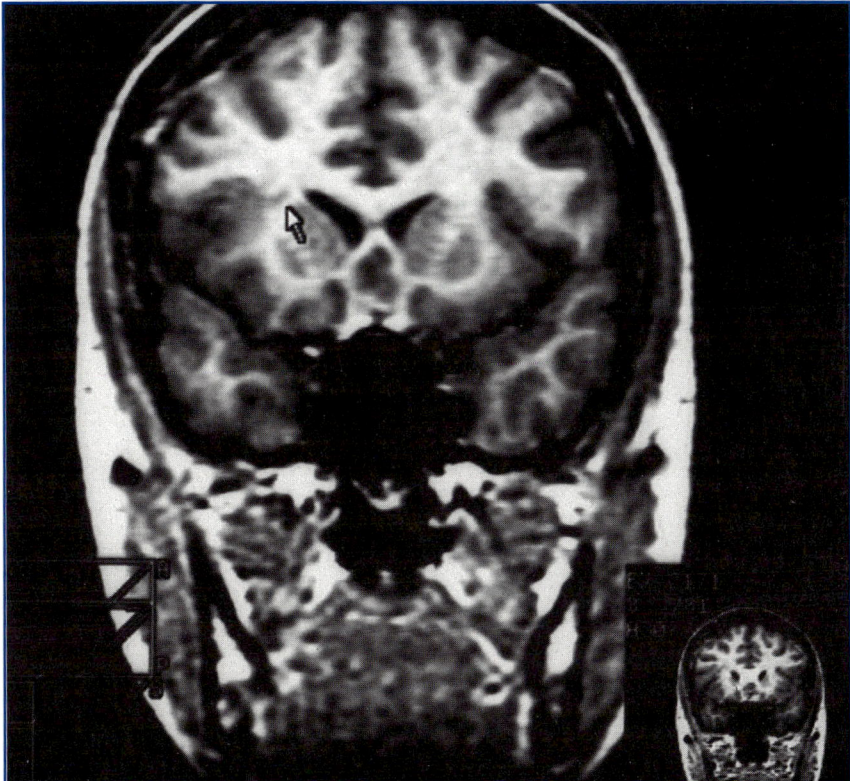

**Figure 16.** *MRI scan showing focal cortical dysplasia. (Courtesy of Dr Sanjay Sisodiya).*

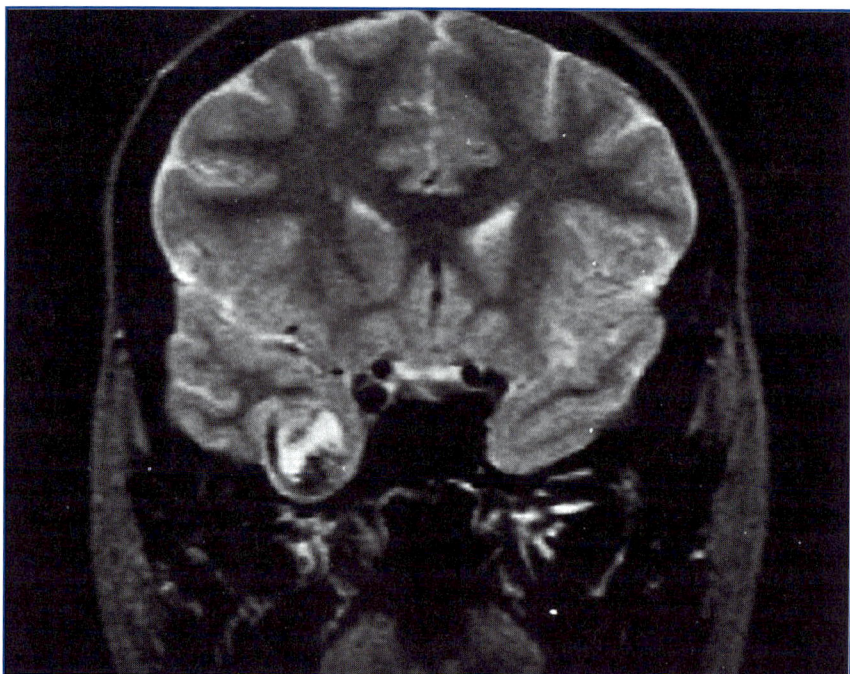

**Figure 17.** *MRI scan showing dysembryoplastic neuroepithelial tumour. (Courtesy of Dr Sanjay Sisodiya).*

### 4.21 What is the association between cortical dysplasias and epilepsy ?

**major cause of chronic epilepsy** *Cortical dysplasias are increasingly being recognised as a major cause of chronic epilepsy.* It has been estimated that at post-mortem examination, cortical dysplasias are found in 25-60% of the brains of patients with epilepsy, compared with 8% of control brains. The majority of these patients had been classified as having cryptogenic epilepsy.

Epilepsy associated with cortical dysplasias often presents in the first decade of life but may be delayed as late as the second decade or even beyond. Except when major abnormalities are present, the intellectual development of patients is usually within the normal range. Many patients with cortical dysplasias give a history of other factors which may have contributed to the development of epilepsy and some people with such lesions never develop epilepsy; it may be that a second insult is required to trigger the seizures in a proportion of cases.

Seizures are usually partial but some patients have only generalised seizures. Response to antiepileptic drug treatment is very variable. Patients with dysembryoplastic neuroepithelial tumours may benefit from surgery.

### 4.22 What is hippocampal sclerosis ?

*Hippocampal sclerosis* (also known as Ammon's horn sclerosis, temporal horn sclerosis or mesial temporal sclerosis) *is the most common lesion identified in pathological specimens of patients with temporal lobe epilepsy who have undergone temporal lobectomy*. It consists of atrophic changes with a variable degree of cell loss and gliosis involving part or the whole of the hippocampus. It is usually unilateral and can be identified by high resolution magnetic resonance imaging (Figure 18). Minor asymmetry of the hippocampi which may suggest sclerosis in the smaller hippocampus is difficult to determine by visual inspection, but can be quantified using MRI-assisted volumetric measurement. Temporal lobe epilepsy with hippocampal sclerosis is strongly associated with a history of prolonged febrile convulsions in childhood.

*most common lesion in patients with temporal lobe epilepsy*

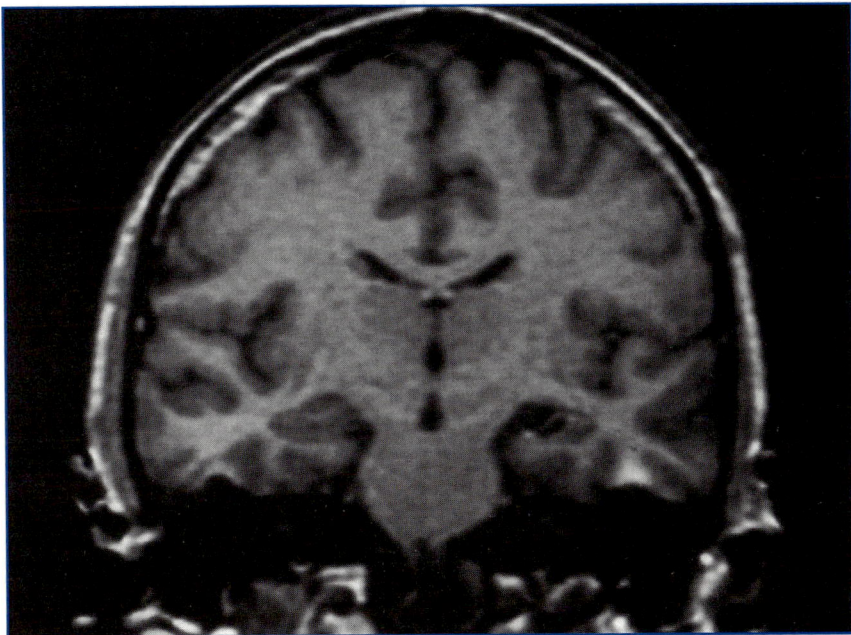

**Figure 18.** *MRI scan showing hippocampal sclerosis. (Courtesy of Dr Sanjay Sisodiya).*

### 4.23 What is the relationship between hippocampal sclerosis and epilepsy?

This ongoing controversy in the epilepsy world questions whether hippocampal sclerosis results from epileptic activity, or whether it precedes the epileptic condition and represents the cause of the seizures. There are some indications that prolonged febrile convulsions in childhood may cause hipppocampal damage and the subsequent development of temporal lobe epilepsy, but this has not yet been proven conclusively. *There is, however, no doubt about the link between severe intractable temporal lobe seizures and hippocampal sclerosis*. Resection of the atrophic area, when possible, is associated with a very good surgical outcome with complete seizure control in over 70% of cases.

### 4.24 Which intrauterine conditions cause seizures ?

**conditions which result in brain damage or malformation**

*Conditions that affect the child while still in the mother's womb may cause epilepsy* as a result of brain damage or malformation. Intrauterine infections (see above) are an example of this, as is erythroblastosis foetalis, an uncommon disease caused by incompatibility between the blood of the foetus and the mother. Cortical dysplasias are also thought to be caused during the intrauterine period (see above).

### 4.25 Which drugs cause seizures?

A number of drugs have been associated with the precipitation of seizures in patients with epilepsy. Most of these drugs may also trigger situation-related seizures in individuals with a low seizure threshold. Examples of such drugs include some antidepressants, antibiotics, anaesthetic agents, antimalarial drugs, beta-blockers, bronchodilators, chemotherapeutic agents, iodinated contrast media and neuroleptic agents. Some recreational drugs such as alcohol, amphetamine and cocaine are also associated with seizures.

### 4.26 Which systemic diseases cause epileptic seizures ?

**epileptic seizures may complicate systemic diseases**

*Epileptic seizures may complicate many systemic diseases, usually as a result of metabolic disturbances*. Any conditions which cause imbalance in the extracellular distribution of sodium, potassium, calcium, magnesium or phosphate have the potential to produce seizures. Hypoglycaemia occurring either in patients taking insulin or other hypoglycaemic agents, or in patients with insulinoma may also present in this way. Other conditions which may be complicated by seizures include acute liver failure, eclampsia, and both acute and chronic renal failure. In the majority of cases, however, these are acute symptomatic attacks and therefore do not constitute epilepsy even if they are recurrent.

### 4.27 What is reflex epilepsy ?

When there is a clear-cut precipitant for epileptic seizures in a given patient, and if seizures only occur as a result of the triggering factor, the condition is referred to as reflex epilepsy. The most common reflex seizures are photically-induced. About 50% of patients with photosensitivity will only have seizures as a response to visual stimuli. Other rarer forms of reflex epilepsy include reading epilepsy, writing epilepsy, startle-induced seizures, arithmetic-induced seizures and musicogenic seizures.

Patients who have seizures precipitated by a particular stimulus but who also have spontaneous seizures should not be classified as having reflex epilepsy.

### 4.28 What is photosensitivity?

In people with idiopathic generalised epilepsy, photosensitivity is a common finding. *Patients with a photosensitive response account for about 2-3% of all people with epilepsy, the proportion being higher in patients aged between 5 and 19 years.* The trait is genetically determined, and may be asymptomatic throughout or present as a medical problem because of epileptic seizures.

**photosensitive responses account for 2-3% of all people with epilepsy**

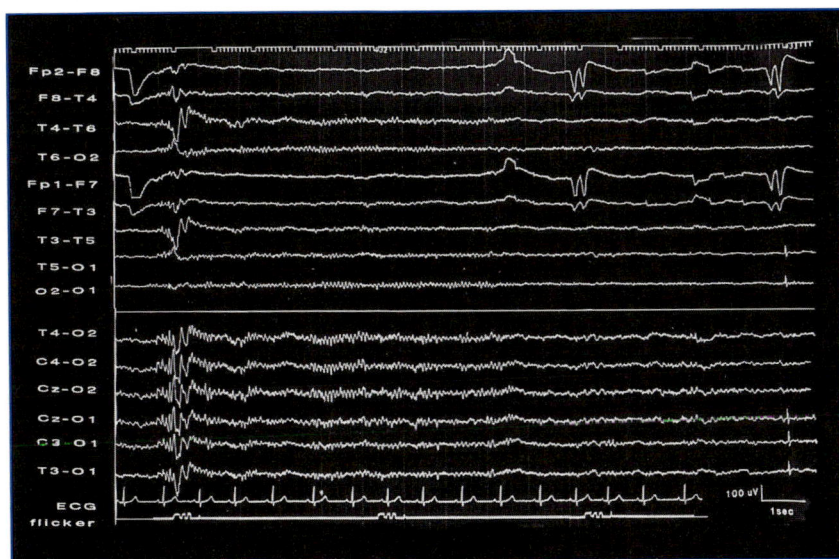

**Figure 19.** *EEG illustrating photosensitivity. (Courtesy of Dr Li Li Min).*

It may only be detected by an EEG (Figure 19) although it should be suspected in patients giving an history of seizures precipitated by flashing lights. Potential precipitants of seizures in photosensitive patients include lights from natural sources such as sunlight passing through trees in a road or reflection in an aquatic surface, or from artificial sources like flashing lights, computer or television screens. *There is no evidence to suggest that flashing lights cause the development of the photosensitive trait, merely that it can trigger seizures in people harbouring this trait.* Photosensitivity is a clinically heterogeneous phenomenon, and photosensitive subjects show wide variation in their susceptibility to seizures.

**no evidence that flashing lights cause photosensitive trait**

### 4.29  What is catamenial epilepsy?

Catamenial epilepsy is the term used to describe seizures occurring in women in association with the menstrual period (either immediately preceding or during menstruation). Suggested causes include hormonal imbalance, water retention and electrolyte disturbances associated with menses. Catamenial epilepsy is discussed further in Chapter 9.

### 4.30  When should epilepsy be termed cryptogenic?

**no putative aetiology is identified**

*The term "cryptogenic epilepsy" is used when no putative aetiology is identified for what is presumed to be a symptomatic or acquired epileptic condition.* Currently about 40% of patients do not have an identifiable cause for their seizures but this proportion is rapidly decreasing as advances in neuroimaging, particularly in magnetic resonance imaging, are made.

The term cryptogenic epilepsy is sometimes used interchangeably with idiopathic epilepsy. This should be avoided, however, as the term idiopathic epilepsy should be reserved for those inherited conditions in which seizures occur as the only manifestation of the disorder.

# CHAPTER 5

## THE PATHOPHYSIOLOGY OF EPILEPSY

### 5.1 What is the pathognomonic lesion of epilepsy?

*Epilepsy differs from most neurological conditions in having no pathognomonic lesion.* Epileptic seizures which are associated with structural abnormalities, however, may have histopathological findings (such as heterotopias or vascular lesions) which are pathognomonic for that condition, rather than for the epilepsy itself. No specific histopathological or histochemical abnormality has yet been identified which is associated with the potential to cause epileptic discharges.

**no pathognomonic lesion**

At the neuronal level, a variety of different electrical or chemical stimuli can lead to the development of seizures in a normal brain. *The hallmark of epilepsy, regardless of the type or aetiology, is a rather rhythmic and repetitive hypersynchronous discharge of neurons, either localised to a particular area of the cerebral cortex or generalised throughout the cortex.* This can usually be demonstrated on an EEG. Despite this, no unifying theory for all aspects of human epileptogenesis has yet been advanced. It is likely that several different pathophysiological mechanisms are responsible for the onset, maintenance and spread of seizures, and these may vary according to the type of epileptic disorder.

**rhythmic and repetitive hypersynchronus discharge of neurons**

A large number of studies using experimental models of epilepsy and functional studies of the brain in vivo using positron emission tomography (PET) and magnetic resonance imaging are being carried out at the present time. It is hoped that enough evidence will eventually emerge to provide a better understanding of the pathophysiology and biochemistry of human epileptogenesis.

### 5.2 What are experimental models of epilepsy ?

Experimental models of epilepsy are standardised methods for producing epilepsy in experimental animals. They are classified into acute and chronic models. The former refers to models which are based on the systemic administration or topical application of convulsant materials or sudden insults such as electrical stimulation which will induce epileptic seizures. Chronic models are based on seizures occurring spontaneously in animals (such as baboons, gerbils and beagle dogs) inbred to produce a genetic predisposition to epilepsy or caused by permanent structural lesions or the repetitive electrical stimulation of areas of the brain.

### 5.3 Can the findings of animal models be extrapolated to human epilepsy ?

**electro-physiological similarities between the animal models and human epilepsy**

Most of what is assumed about human epileptogenesis is extrapolated from research carried out in experimental animal models of epilepsy. These models have never been properly validated and the relevance of these results to human epilepsy is therefore difficult to assess. *There are, however, some electrophysiological similarities between the animal models and human epilepsy*, and some findings from animal models have been confirmed in vivo. This gives some credence to the assumption that findings from these models can be applied to human epilepsy.

### 5.4 What is the role of neurotransmitters in the genesis of epilepsy?

Neurons are interconnected in a complex network in which each individual neuron is linked through synapses with hundreds of others. *A small electrical discharge in a neuron causes the release of a neurotransmitter substance at the synaptic level, thus enabling communication between neurons*. Neurotransmitters are of two types: inhibitory and excitatory.

**enables communication between neurons**

A discharging neuron may thus either excite or inhibit neurons associated with it. An excited neuron will activate the next neuron whereas an inhibited neuron will not. In this manner, information is transmitted throughout the central nervous system.

A whole array of neurotransmitters seem to exist and it is quite possible that some have not yet been identified. *The most important known inhibitory neurotransmitter is gamma-amino-butyric acid (GABA) of which several forms have already been recognised*. Excitatory transmission seems to be dependent on amino acids, of which glutamate and aspartate are the most well-known at this stage. It is possible that either a lack or an excess of neurotransmitters of either category may play a part in the disruption of the processes of neuronal transmission and thus lead to epileptic seizures.

**gamma-amino butyric acid**

## 5.5  How does an epileptic seizure start?

A normal neuron discharges repetitively at a low baseline frequency and
it is the integrated electrical activity generated by the neurons of the
superficial layers of the cortex which is recorded in a normal EEG.  If
neurons are damaged or suffer a chemical or metabolic insult, a change in
the pattern of discharges may develop.  In the case of *partial epilepsy,
regular low frequency discharges are replaced by bursts of high frequency
discharges usually followed by periods of inactivity*.  A single neuron
discharging in an abnormal manner is usually of no clinical significance:
it is only when a whole population of neurons discharge synchronously
in an abnormal way that an epileptic seizure may be triggered.  Little is
known about the precise mechanisms which lead to this synchronisation
and consequently to seizure onset.  The abnormal discharge may remain
localised or it may spread to adjacent areas recruiting more neurons as it
spreads.  It may also generalise throughout the brain via cortical and
subcortical routes including callosal and thalamocortical pathways.  The
area from which the abnormal discharge originates is known as the
epileptic focus.

*In the idiopathic generalised absences the mechanisms are even less
understood but they are probably different*.  The discharges are thought to
arise from or be modulated by the thalamus rather than from the cerebral
cortex and the way they spread is also likely to be different.

**bursts of high frequency discharges**

## 5.6  Why are seizures self-limited?

It is not known why epileptic seizures cease spontaneously in the vast
majority of cases.  It is likely that inhibitory substances are released in the
cortex and terminate the seizure.  Recent speculation has centred on the
role of endogenous opioids in such a process.

## 5.7  Does ictal activity cause brain damage?

*Another controversial area in epilepsy is whether seizure activity may
itself cause neuronal damage or functional changes*.  It has been
suggested that chronic epileptic discharges may lead to secondary
epileptogenesis (kindling).  Evidence for this in some experimental models
of partial seizures is convincing but similar evidence is lacking in humans,
in whom the hypothesis is difficult to test.

**chronic epileptic discharges may lead to secondary epileptogenesis**

*It is thought that short, uncomplicated seizures cause no permanent or progressive neurological dysfunction in humans.* Prolonged generalised tonic clonic status epilepticus is associated with a high neurological morbidity and may result in permanent brain damage. It is, however, probable that this is at least in part due to systemic factors such as hypoperfusion, hypoxia, acidosis and other metabolic disturbances associated with status.

# CHAPTER 6

## THE DIAGNOSIS AND INVESTIGATION OF EPILEPSY

### 6.1 How is the diagnosis of epilepsy made?

*The diagnosis of epilepsy is essentially clinical, and rests on the description of the seizure provided by the patient and an eye-witness.* The report of the eye-witness is of great importance, especially if there is any impairment of consciousness during the seizure.  An attempt should be made at the same time to identify any condition which could cause epileptic seizures, and categorise the seizure according to the classifications of the International League Against Epilepsy.

**clinical diagnosis**

Issues which should be particularly addressed include the nature of the aura, if present; the ictal manifestations themselves; and the presence or absence of post-ictal confusion, drowsiness, or headache. *Precipitating factors should be addressed.  A full medical (including neurological) history should be taken in addition to details of previous psychiatric problems, and a family history.* The patient should be asked particularly whether he or she has ever had febrile convulsions, significant head injury, encephalitis or meningitis, and whether the birth was normal.

**detailed medical history**

### 6.2 With what conditions may epilepsy be confused?

There are many disorders involving alteration of consciousness, or focal neurological symptoms, which may be confused with epileptic seizures; these are summarised in Table 4.  *The conditions most commonly mistaken for epileptic seizures are syncope and pseudoseizures.*

**syncope and pseudoseizures**

#### Syncope

Syncope may be due to a number of causes, including strong emotion, prolonged standing, particularly if the ambient temperature is hot, cardiac arrhythmias, coughing, and hypovolaemia.  Except in those cases caused by cardiac arrhythmias, it rarely occurs in patients who are recumbent.

It is almost invariably preceded by a warning in which the patient feels faint and sometimes sick, the vision becomes blurred, and hearing may be lost. To an observer, the patient appears pale, and may sweat profusely. Consciousness is then usually lost and the patient falls to the floor. Quick recovery occurs provided the patient is not raised to an upright position. Incontinence and injury are rare. If the patient is raised, there may be some jerking of the limbs or even a tonic clonic seizure. Afterwards, the patient may feel nauseated and shaky but not confused or drowsy. *The features of cardiac syncope can often differ* in that the patient may have no warning, and does not necessarily recover on lying down.

**Table 4.** *Conditions which may be confused with epilepsy.*

| | |
|---|---|
| Syncope | Movement disorders |
| Pseudoseizures | Narcolepsy |
| Panic attacks | Transient ischaemic attacks |
| Hyperventilation | Migraine |
| Episodic dyscontrol syndrome | Transient global amnesia |
| Breath-holding attacks | Hypoglycaemia |
| Night terrors | Vertigo |
| Day-dreaming | |

**Pseudoseizures**

These are sometimes termed psychogenic seizures, although some authors use the latter term to describe genuine epileptic seizures induced by the patient at will, for example, by fluttering the eyelids in the case of photosensitive epilepsy. Other terms used to describe this condition are non-epileptic attack disorder (NEAD) and hysterical seizures. *It is common experience in specialised centres that around 20% of patients admitted to hospital with a diagnosis of intractable epilepsy do not have epileptic seizures.* However, pseudoseizures also occur not infrequently in people with epilepsy.

**more common in women** *Pseudoseizures are more common in women.* They may have a past or family history of psychiatric disorder, sometimes including unexplained neurological dysfunction or previous attempted suicide. The attacks tend to start in the teens or twenties, and do not respond to the introduction of antiepileptic drugs, unlike genuine epileptic seizures. If the attacks have the appearance of generalised tonic clonic seizures, serial measurements of serum prolactin levels after a seizure may help in the differentiation from genuine epileptic attacks. Pseudostatus epilepticus may also occur in patients with pseudoseizures, who are thus at risk of receiving large doses of antiepileptic medication even to the extent that assisted ventilation may be required, with all the attendant hazards.

## Panic attacks

*Panic attacks are common in people with anxiety states*. The patient feels anxious, and this feeling is accompanied by such physical symptoms as palpitations, dyspnoea, sweating, trembling, and abdominal discomfort. Usually it is possible to distinguish such attacks from the history, but occasionally seizures of temporal lobe origin may have similar symptomatology.

## Hyperventilation

This is another common disorder which is not infrequently confused with epilepsy. *Attacks usually occur during periods of stress*. Hyperventilation causes a feeling of dizziness and sometimes even altered awareness or loss of consciousness. The patient may also complain of chest pain, dyspnoea, blurred vision, paraesthesias, muscle cramps and fatigue.

**periods of stress**

## Episodic dyscontrol syndrome

*Rage attacks, often occurring apparently out of character, are sometimes attributed to epilepsy*. In practice however, rage occurring in the context of epileptic seizures is rare, unprovoked, and usually undirected.

## Breath-holding attacks

*These occur in children, usually under the age of six years, and are commonly mistaken for seizures*, although if witnessed, diagnosis should be possible from the history of precipitating factors. Cyanotic breath-holding attacks occur when the child is frustrated or angry. A period of crying is followed by the cessation of breathing. Cyanosis follows and the child becomes limp and unresponsive; sometimes trembling or a few clonic movements occur. Unresponsiveness usually persists for about two

**occur in younger children**

minutes and is followed by rapid recovery. Pallid breath-holding attacks often follow minor head-trauma. The child may not cry, but abruptly loses consciousness and becomes limp. Clonic movements are common as a result of cerebral hypoxia, but recovery is fairly rapid.

### Day-dreaming

*Innocent day-dreaming may occasionally be mistaken for true absence attacks*, but can be distinguished by the fact that the child can be easily alerted, and by the absence of postural changes or automatisms.

### Sleep phenomena

*There are several sleep phenomena which may be confused with epileptic seizures*. Sleep-walking is common in children, and is characterised by automatic behaviour (which does not always involve the patient getting out of bed) during non-REM sleep. Night-terrors are also common in children and likewise occur in deep slow-wave sleep. The child suddenly sits up, crying or screaming, sweating and with dilated pupils. Eventually the child calms down and normal sleep is resumed. Afterwards however, there is amnesia for the attack. It is less common for nightmares to be mistaken for seizures. *Hypnic jerks occur in the majority of people from time to time*, and take the form of a single jerk occurring in the early stages of sleep, often accompanied by a falling sensation and causing awakening. Periodic movements of sleep occur in later life and are characterised by the presence of repetitive rhythmic leg movements, often with dorsiflexion of the foot and extension of the toes. Sleep apnoea may rarely also be mistaken for epilepsy. Paroxysmal nocturnal dystonias, which at one time were considered to be an uncommon movement disorder of sleep, are now recognised to be due to frontal lobe seizures.

*Narcolepsy is a condition in which sudden irresistible attacks of daytime sleepiness occur*. Cataplexy is characterised by sudden falls as a result of postural tone loss; either type of attack may occasionally be confused with epileptic seizures.

**may be confused with epileptic seizures**

## Migraine

*There are several reasons why migraine attacks may be confused with epileptic seizures*. Syncope may occur during the course of migraine, particularly when vomiting occurs. Basilar migraine may present with loss of consciousness, often in association with other symptoms and followed by headache, causing confusion with epileptic seizures. The acompanying brainstem symptoms and a family history of migraine may help in their differentiation. *Migraine preceded by visual or sensory disturbances may also be mistaken for partial epilepsies*. It should be noted that interictal paroxysmal EEG phenomena may be seen in migraine.

**migraine preceded by visual or sensory disturbances**

## Transient ischaemic attacks

Transient ischaemic attacks may produce weakness and sensory symptoms; it is the latter which usually cause confusion with epileptic seizures. *Transient ischaemic attacks usually last longer than epileptic seizures, and there is rarely loss of consciousness*. Sensory phenomena in epilepsy may spread in the manner of a Jacksonian march. This is not usually the case in transient ischaemic attacks.

**last longer than epileptic seizures**

## Transient global amnesia

Transient global amnesia is a condition usually occurring in middle-aged or older people. Most often this occurs as an isolated episode lasting several hours, in which the patient is unable to remember. He or she remains alert and communicative throughout this period, but may repeatedly ask the same question. *Except for amnesia, during of the episode, recovery afterwards is complete.* The cause of transient global amnesia remains unclear. Migraine, epilepsy and cerebrovascular disease have been suggested, but it is thought that only a small minority of patients with such symptoms have epilepsy, and in these, the attacks are usually short-lived and recurrent.

## Movement disorders

A variety of movement disorders may on occasion be mistaken for seizures, although the distinction is not usually difficult. *Tics and chorea may sometimes be confused with myoclonus*. Paroxysmal choreoathetosis is a familial disorder characterised by repeated episodes of dystonia or

**tics and chorea may be confused with myoclonus**

choreoathetosis, unaccompanied by loss of consciousness. Despite the absence of ictal EEG abnormalities, the condition often responds to antiepileptic medication. In paroxysmal kinesigenic choreoathetosis the attacks, which are short-lived, are precipitated by sudden movement. Tonic spasms similar to those seen in paroxysmal chorea are also sometimes seen in multiple sclerosis.

**paroxysmal familial ataxia is an inherited condition**

*Paroxysmal familial ataxia is an inherited condition* in which episodes of ataxia lasting up to 30 minutes may occur, without other accompaniments. *It has been reported in people of Mediterranean origin*, and it is important to recognise since it may have an excellent response to acetazolamide.

### Hypoglycaemia

This is an uncommon condition affecting people with diabetes, and in particular, those taking insulin or oral hypoglycaemic agents. Occasionally however, it is due to insulinoma. Hypoglycaemia normally first produces autonomic changes, including pallor, sweating, and tachycardia, and these may be recognised by the patient who can then take appropriate action. If autonomic changes do not occur, or if there is no warning, coma ensues, and genuine seizures may eventually supervene.

### Vertigo

**misdiagnosed as epilepsy**

*Vertigo has many causes, but is often paroxysmal, and as a result, is sometimes misdiagnosed as epilepsy*. Very occasionally, vertigo may itself be a symptom of an epileptic seizure, particularly in the case of parietal lobe epilepsy.

### 6.3 Are there any particular signs which should be sought in the examination of patients with epilepsy?

**focal neurological deficits should be sought**

*All patients developing seizures should have a complete general and neurological examination*. Specific signs which should be checked include the presence of any cutaneous stigmata which may indicate the cause of the epilepsy (café au lait spots, adenoma sebaceum, or trigeminal capillary haemangiomas, suggesting the possibility of neurofibromatosis, tuberous sclerosis, and Sturge-Weber syndrome respectively). *Focal neurological deficits suggesting the presence of a structural lesion should be assiduously sought*. Abnormalities may be subtle, for example, impairment

of fine finger movements. The patient should also be examined for any
evidence of hemiatrophy, indicating a cerebral lesion occurring early in life.

## 6.4 Which patients, if any, require investigation after a single seizure?

The aims of investigation are to increase diagnostic accuracy and clarify the
seizure type, and  most importantly to identify the cause of the seizures.  An
indication of prognosis may also be obtained if a specific cause or epilepsy
syndrome, such as benign epilepsy of childhood with centrotemporal spikes,
is identified.  It has been argued that seizures occurring as a result of tumour
or other sinister cause are likely to recur, and that investigation may be
deferred until the occurrence of a second seizure. However, the identification
of an underlying cause or syndrome may have implications for prognosis
or treatment, and *we recommend investigation at an early stage in all
patients developing seizures*.

**investigation of
seizures at
an early stage**

## 6.5 Which investigations should be performed in patients developing seizures?

As has been stated above, *the diagnosis of epilepsy is clinical, and depends
mainly on the description of the attack*.  However, the finding of obvious
epileptic abnormalities in the EEG lends weight to the diagnosis, and the
seizure type may also be clarified.  The use of the EEG is described in
more detail below.

**epileptic
abnormalities in
the EEG**

*The history and examination not infrequently give a clue to aetiology,*
particularly in the case of acute symptomatic or situation-related seizures
(seizures occurring in the context of a metabolic disturbance, drugs, or other
acute insult to the brain, such as head injury, stroke or infection).  Seizures
can occur with disorders of sodium, calcium, magnesium, and glucose
metabolism, in renal failure and acute hepatic failure, and occasionally with
thyroid disease.  Biochemical tests for these disorders, in addition to full
blood count, erythrocyte sedimentation rate (ESR), and syphilis serology,
should be performed as clinically indicated.  However, routine screening in
otherwise fit people has a low yield.

Blackouts or dizzy spells due to cardiac arrhythmias may be confused with
seizures. An electrocardiogram or 24 hour cardiac monitoring should be
performed where appropriate, particularly in the elderly.

**Table 5.** *Causes of neonatal seizures.*

> Birth asphyxia
> Infection
> Metabolic disorders (including hypoglycaemia, hypocalcaemia, pyridoxine deficiency)
> Intracranial haemorrhage
> Maternal drug use
> Benign idiopathic neonatal convulsions ("fifth day fits")
> Benign familial neonatal convulsions
> Other

In children, the possibility of inborn errors of metabolism should be considered (Table 5). Special investigation is only necessary when there are specific features to suggest such a condition, and should be tailored according to the clinical picture.

*birth asphyxia is considered the largest single cause of neonatal seizures*

The major causes of neonatal seizures are shown in Table 5. The proportion of seizures due to each cause has differed in various studies, but *the largest single cause of neonatal seizures* (30-50%) *is considered to be birth asphyxia*. However, in some surveys up to one third of neonatal seizures have been benign idiopathic neonatal convulsions ("fifth-day fits"). The cause of the seizures may be suggested by the history and examination, and investigations need to be tailored to the individual infant.

**6.6 How does an EEG help in making the diagnosis of epilepsy?**

*The diagnosis of epilepsy can neither be made nor refuted on the basis of an interictal EEG, though epileptic abnormalities make the diagnosis more likely.* Approximately 35% of patients with epilepsy show interictal epileptiform activity in all routine waking recordings, 15% do not show interictal epileptiform abnormalities even after multiple EEGs, and the remainder (50-55%) show epileptiform activity in some but not all recordings.

Less than 1% of normal subjects, with no clinical evidence of epilepsy and without other cerebral disease, have focal or generalised spike or polyspike and wave abnormalities on the EEG, although between 10 and 15% of the population may have minor non-specific abnormalities. People undergoing EEG examinations because of other complaints, but without clinical evidence of seizures, have an incidence of epileptiform abnormalities of 2-3%, as do those taking major tranquillisers or antidepressants. In those with learning difficulties the incidence may be as high as 30%.

### 6.7  If the initial EEG is normal, are there other investigations which may be helpful in making the diagnosis?

If epilepsy is suggested clinically, corroborative evidence may be derived from an EEG obtained during sleep (either drug-induced or following sleep deprivation), since interictal epileptiform activity, particularly that associated with partial epilepsy, is often increased during drowsiness and light sleep. *In patients having frequent attacks, prolonged EEG with video-monitoring may allow the recording of an ictal event and confirm the diagnosis.* However, it should be noted that not all cortical spikes are recorded by scalp EEG, and hence an absence of ictal change in the EEG does not rule out the possibility of epilepsy. This is particularly the case for simple partial seizures, seizures arising in the mesial or orbital frontal regions, and seizures in which the only manifestation is a visceral aura.

**prolonged EEG with video-monitoring may allow the recording of an ictal event**

### 6.8  How can the EEG help to clarify the seizure type?

The EEG in the generalised epilepsies typically shows the presence of generalised epileptiform discharges, often of the spike and wave variety, although polyspike activity is also not uncommon. *Typical absence epilepsy (formerly known as "petit mal" epilepsy) is characterised by 3 per second spike and wave activity.* Such activity can often be brought out during hyperventilation. In juvenile myoclonic epilepsy, photosensitivity (the development of epileptic activity in response to photic stimulation) is common, while the ictal and interictal EEG show generalised irregular spike and slow wave discharges.

**typical absence epilepsy can be characterised**

It is often difficult to distinguish primary generalised seizures from secondarily generalised seizures on a clinical basis, particularly if the spread of seizure activity in the partial epilepsy occurs quickly so that no aura is experienced. *An ictal EEG may demonstrate the partial onset of such seizures, while interictal EEGs may also raise this possibility by demonstrating focal epileptiform activity.* However, caution is needed in the interpretation of the interictal EEG since both partial and generalised epileptic activity may occur in the same patient.

**ictal and interictal EEG issues**

Apart from its use in identifying the seizure focus in some patients with symptomatic epilepsy (ie, epilepsy secondary to a known cause), the EEG may also show typical features in idiopathic partial epilepsies such as benign epilepsy of childhood with centrotemporal spikes, and benign epilepsy of childhood with occipital paroxysms, rendering further investigation unnecessary in the presence of a typical clinical history.

### 6.9 Does prolonged EEG with video-monitoring have any role other than the diagnosis of epilepsy?

In addition to clarifying the diagnosis of epilepsy in some patients, prolonged EEG with video-monitoring plays a very important role in the evaluation of patients being considered for surgical treatment of their epilepsy. It allows close examination of the clinical features of the seizure, and the recording should include questioning of the patient during and after the seizure to assess responsiveness, verbal and memory function. Evaluation for post-ictal paresis should also be carried out. The clinical features may themselves permit accurate localisation of the seizure **careful** discharge, with the EEG providing further information about the site of **interpretation** onset. *Caution is needed in the interpretation of both clinical and EEG* **of clinical** *features however, since false localisation may occur.* Where doubt about **and EEG** the site of the epileptic focus remains after prolonged EEG with video- **features** monitoring with scalp electrodes, recording with depth electrodes may be necessary.

### 6.10 Is an EEG indicated prior to discontinuation of medication?

**use of the** There has been controversy as to whether interictal epileptiform activity is **EEG in** of prognostic significance with regard to recurrence of seizures in patients **predicting** stopping antiepileptic medication. *The available evidence suggests that in* **subsequent** *adults, the EEG is of little help in predicting subsequent relapse, while in* **relapse** *children, an active interictal epileptiform disturbance probably indicates a slight increase in the risk of recurrent seizures.*

### 6.11 When should a CT scan be performed?

**usefulness of** *In adults the chance of finding a structural lesion as a cause of seizures is* **the CT scan or** *greater than in children, and either a CT scan, or preferably an MRI scan,* **MRI scan in** *should be performed in almost every case.* This is particularly true where **adult diagnosis** the seizures are focal, where neurological abnormalities are found on examination, or where there is EEG evidence of a focal abnormality. Children with clinically obvious primary generalised epilepsy do not require neuroimaging, but neuroimaging is warranted in most children with partial seizures except where these clearly conform to a "benign" syndrome such as benign epilepsy of childhood with centrotemporal spikes. CT scanning is justified in any child less than one year old presenting with epileptic seizures, since structural lesions are often present, most idiopathic epilepsies starting after this age.

## 6.12 Does an MRI scan have advantages over a CT scan in people with epilepsy?

*MRI scans have a number of advantages over CT scans.* Certain abnormalities which may not be shown on CT scan because they are isodense with brain may be demonstrated by MRI scan: these include demyelinating lesions, encephalitis, and some low-grade gliomas. Neuronal migration disorders are one cause of seizures which may sometimes be apparent on CT scan but most often are only visualised by MRI. Mesial temporal sclerosis may also be demonstrated by MRI, and volumetric measurements can be used to demonstrate atrophy of the amygdala and hippocampus, which are often associated with temporal lobe epilepsy. Another advantage of magnetic resonance imaging is that it does not involve ionising radiation, and is hence thought not to constitute a biological hazard. Calcification (which may occur in oligodendrogliomas or cavernous angiomas) is better demonstrated by CT scanning.

**advantage of the MRI**

## 6.13 When are SPECT and PET scanning indicated?

*The main use of SPECT (single photon emission computed tomography) and PET (positron emission tomography) in epilepsy is in pre-operative evaluation.* PET provides better resolution than SPECT scanning but requires a cyclotron on site since the isotopes used have very short half-lives. Interictally, unilaterally reduced cerebral glucose metabolism, measured using 18-F-2-deoxyglucose (FDG) is seen in 70-80% of patients with complex partial seizures (Figure 20) usually over the temporal lobe. Ictal FDG-PET studies are rarely obtained, but may show increased glucose metabolism at the site of the epileptic focus. Cerebral blood flow may also be measured using $^{15}O$ labelled gases (by inhalation) or water (by injection) and give similar results to those obtained with FDG-PET,

**pre-operative evaluation**

although the methods may not be as sensitive. *SPECT scanning* does not require an on-site cyclotron and *is less expensive than PET*. It provides similar information to that obtained for cerebral blood flow measurements with PET, but the resolution is not as good and the method is less sensitive (about 50% of patients with focal seizures having reduced interictal cerebral blood flow). However, in 15-20% of patients lateralisation does not concur with the EEG results. The advantage of SPECT over PET scanning is that ictal scans can be obtained because the half-lives of the isotopes are longer, increased blood flow being shown on the side of the EEG focus in 65-90% of patients.

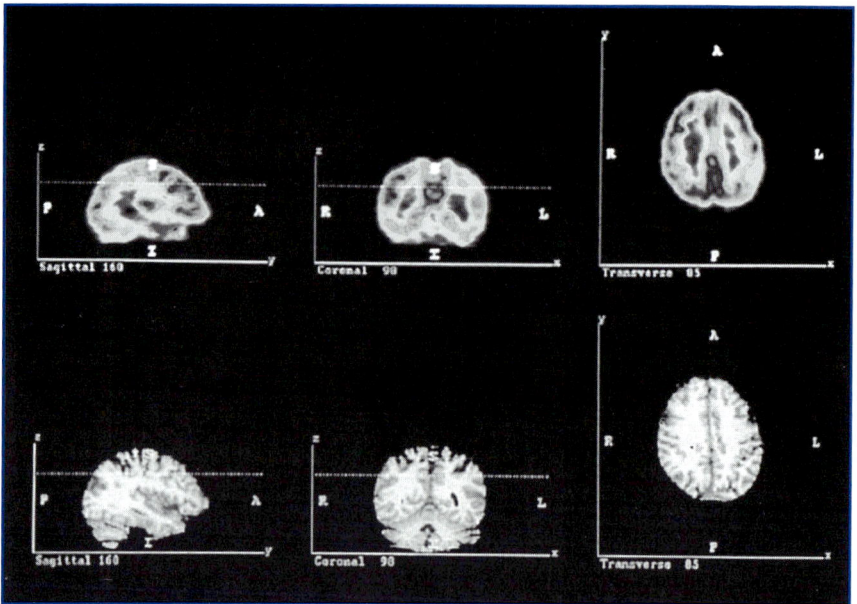

**Figure 20.** *FDG-PET scan showing L posterior hemisphere hypometabolism superimposed on MRI. (Courtsey of Dr John Duncan).*

### 6.14 When is neuropsychological testing appropriate?

the risk of
psychological
problems

*People with epilepsy may be at risk of psychological problems for a variety of reasons.* The epilepsy may produce problems of adjustment, and particularly in young children parental overprotection may impair social development. It seems likely that seizures themselves may cause brain damage if they are very prolonged or frequent. Subclinical epileptic discharges can cause transient cognitive defects and if the epilepsy is symptomatic, the underlying lesion may also be associated with problems of cognition.  The adverse effect of antiepileptic drugs on mental functioning has become much more widely recognised in recent years. It could therefore be argued that neuropsychological assessment is appropriate in most people developing epilepsy.  In practice, such assessment is not often performed and may not be readily available. Since, in the majority of people developing epilepsy, seizures are readily controlled with monotherapy using modern drugs, it would seem reasonable to reserve such assessment for people who have obvious or possible psychological or learning difficulties, and those whose seizures are intractable, particularly if surgery is contemplated.

# CHAPTER 7

# THE MEDICAL TREATMENT OF EPILEPSY

### 7.1 When should treatment for epilepsy be started?

*The first requirement before antiepileptic medication is started is that the patient should have had confirmed epileptic seizures*. In practice this may be difficult, and it is not uncommon for several months to elapse between the time of the first afebrile seizure and confirmation of the diagnosis of epilepsy.

*The second issue of importance when considering treatment relates to the likelihood of recurrence after a first seizure. This has been estimated at between 27 and 84%.* The differences between the results found by the various studies are largely methodological: in some, patients with a first seizure have been identified only at their first hospital visit, for example, so that patients having an early recurrence (before being seen) would be excluded, while in other studies, most people have received antiepileptic drugs after the initial seizure. Such factors are liable to reduce the apparent rate of recurrence.

*The probability of a second seizure is greatest immediately after the initial event* and falls thereafter. The aetiology of the seizures also influences the chance of recurrence: there is evidence that acute symptomatic seizures (those occurring in the context of an acute insult to the brain, such as stroke or encephalitis, or in association with metabolic derangement or drugs) are less likely to recur than idiopathic seizures or remote symptomatic seizures, while seizures occurring in patients with a neurological deficit present from birth have the highest rate of recurrence. There is controversy about the effect of age at onset of seizures on recurrence.

In Europe, most neurologists do not recommend starting antiepileptic treatment until the occurrence of a second seizure, unless there is a specific factor (such as the presence of a cerebral tumour, or the occurrence of unprovoked status epilepticus at presentation) which makes recurrence very likely. This reduces the chance of people taking

**confirmed epileptic seizures before medication**

**likelihood of recurrence**

**probability of a second seizure**

**specific factors examined**

antiepileptic drugs unnecessarily for long periods of time (the risk of a third seizure after a second has occurred is even greater than the risk of recurrence after a first seizure).

**medical and social considerations**

In the United States, it is often recommended that antiepileptic treatment is started after a first seizure. However, *the decision regarding when to start antiepileptic drugs must be discussed fully with the patient, and must take into account both medical and social considerations*.

The crucial issue of whether, as postulated by Gowers, "...the effect of a convulsion on the nerve centres is such as to render the occurrence of another more easy, to intensify the predisposition that already exists. Thus every fit may be said to be, in part, the result of those that have preceded it, the cause of those which follow it..." remains controversial, and studies are currently under way to try to resolve this issue.

**patient preference for treatment**

A small number of patients have very infrequent seizures, perhaps one every year or two. In these patients the need for treatment from the medical point of view is not great, and some patients prefer not to take medication every day in order to prevent a very occasional event. For others, however, the uncertainty as to when a seizure will occur or the wish to drive mean that they would prefer to take regular medication, and this is a reasonable choice.

*A proportion of patients only experience seizures while asleep, and may prefer not to take medication*. Other factors which should be considered when deciding whether antiepileptic treatment is appropriate include the type of epileptic seizure or syndrome, the likelihood of compliance with treatment, and the presumed aetiology. If a patient has seizures accompanied by a high risk of injury (such as atonic seizures) the need for treatment is greater than for patients with minor simple partial seizures having little effect on everyday life.

**compliance is vital**

Some epilepsy syndromes, such as benign epilepsy of childhood with centrotemporal spikes, have a benign prognosis, and if seizures occur mainly during the night or are infrequent, medication may be unnecessary. Patients in whom seizures are regularly precipitated by alcohol (or its withdrawal) or abuse of drugs are better served by abstinence from the offending agent than by medication, with which they may not be compliant. *Compliance is of particular importance in the treatment of epilepsy, since withdrawal seizures may be precipitated by the abrupt cessation of medication*.

Some patients, such as those with malignant tumours or other progressive **compliance is** neurological conditions, are at higher risk of recurrence and in these **important** patients, medication is usually appropriate after a single seizure.

Patients whose seizures occur in the context of a metabolic disorder or acute insult to the brain, in contrast, are less likely to have a recurrence.

### 7.2 What advice should be given to patients starting treatment for epilepsy?

In some patients, *seizures can be precipitated by certain stimuli*. Examples of such precipitants include excessive alcohol intake, sleep deprivation, flickering lights (such as may occur with television screens, computer games and discotheques), and menstruation.

Avoidance of precipitants where feasible may be helpful, but most of **unprovoked** these patients will nonetheless require medication to control unprovoked **seizures** seizures. It should be stressed that only a few people with epilepsy are photosensitive, while the majority are able to enjoy discotheques and use computer screens without problem.

*The need for medication to be taken regularly should be stressed, and the patient advised of the risk of withdrawal seizures if medication is abruptly withdrawn*. The aims of treatment and the need for it to be **the importance** continued even when seizures are controlled should be fully explained. **of medication** Other issues which should be addressed include possible drug interactions (including the interaction of those drugs causing hepatic enzyme induction with the oral contraceptive pill).

People often ask about the interaction of alcohol with antiepileptic drugs (AEDs). The majority of people are able to take modest amounts of alcohol without problem: they should be advised, however, that the **interaction** sedative effects of some antiepileptic drugs may be enhanced. **with alcohol**

# E PILEPSY

### 7.3 What advice should be given to relatives and carers about the management of seizures?

Convulsive seizures may look frightening, and advice should be given to relatives or carers as to how to cope with them. It should be stressed that the patient is not in pain and will usually have no recollection of the event afterwards, *seizures are generally self-limited, and serious injury is rare*. Attendance at hospital is seldom necessary.

**serious injury is rare**

Patients should be made as comfortable as possible, preferably lying down (they should be eased to the floor if sitting), and the head should be cushioned. Any tight clothing or neckwear should be loosened. During seizures, patients should not be moved, unless they are in a dangerous place, for example in a road, by a fire or hot radiator, at the top of stairs or by the edge of water.

**do not open the patient's mouth**

*No attempt should be made to open the patient's mouth or force anything between the teeth*. If the tongue is bitten during an attack, this almost invariably happens at the beginning, and well-meaning attempts to prevent it or protect the airway in this way usually result in damage. Broken teeth may be inhaled, causing secondary lung damage. When the seizure stops, the patient should be moved into the recovery position.

Partial attacks are usually less dramatic. During automatisms, patients may behave in a confused fashion and should generally be left undisturbed. Gentle restraint may be necessary if the automatism leads to dangerous wandering. Attempts at firm restraint, however, may increase agitation and confusion and provoke aggression.

**no drinks or drugs following an attack . . . offer reassurance**

*No drinks should be given after an attack, nor should extra antiepileptic drugs be given*. Onlookers are often worried that a patient may die during a seizure, but such an occurrence is exceedingly rare. *After a seizure*, it is important to *stay with the patient and offer reassurance* until the confused period has subsided and the patient has recovered fully.

If a seizure persists for more than 10 minutes, if a series of seizures occur, or if the seizure is particularly severe, then intravenous or rectal administration of diazepam is advisable (assuming facilities are available).

### 7.4 How should drug treatment be instituted?

Approximately 60-70% of patients developing epilepsy will have their seizures controlled with monotherapy using a first-line drug and research has shown that in most patients seizure control is optimal with monotherapy, while adverse effects are minimised. Drug interactions and poor compliance are also more likely with polytherapy. However, 10-15% of patients require two drugs for optimal seizure control.

*The patient should be treated initially with a first-line drug appropriate to the seizure-type. The drug is usually started at a low dose, which is gradually increased until either the seizures are controlled, or toxic effects are experienced by the patient.* Some drugs are particularly liable to cause toxic symptoms if the dose is increased too quickly, and every effort should be made to avoid this situation, since it may well make the patient reluctant to continue medication. If the first drug fails to control seizures or is not tolerated, another first-line drug is tried and the previous drug withdrawn.

**initial treatment with first-line drug**

### 7.5 What is the drug of choice in patients with generalised tonic clonic seizures?

*Carbamazepine, sodium valproate and phenytoin are all effective in the treatment of generalised tonic clonic seizures, whether primary or secondarily generalised.* In patients with a mixed generalised seizure disorder (with myoclonus or true absence attacks in addition to generalised tonic clonic seizures, for example), sodium valproate is usually the drug of choice.

**effective drugs in tonic-clonic seizures**

### 7.6 Which other drugs are helpful in the treatment of generalised epileptic seizures?

In patients with *true absence attacks alone, ethosuximide is an effective drug.* The benzodiazephines (such as clonazepam) may be helpful in the treatment of myoclonus.

**true absence attacks**

### 7.7 Which drugs may be used in the treatment of partial seizures?

**medication for partial seizures**

Carbamazepine, phenytoin and sodium valproate are all effective in this respect. *Gabapentin, felbamate, lamotrigine, tiagabine, topiramate and vigabatrin may all be helpful in the management of partial seizures.* Some of these are newer drugs and are as yet only marketed for the treatment of refractory seizures in certain countries.

### 7.8 What is the procedure if the first drug fails?

**reassessing the diagnosis**

*If treatment with a drug appropriate for the suspected seizure type fails in any patient with a new diagnosis of epilepsy, the patient should be reassessed, with particular attention to whether the diagnosis of epilepsy is correct, and whether the seizures have an underlying aetiology which remains to be identified. Enquiries should also be made about*

**check compliance and drug levels**

*compliance with medication, and serum drug levels checked.* Assuming these are satisfactory, another appropriate drug should be commenced, and the initial drug gradually withdrawn.

The dose of the second drug should be titrated in the same manner as the first until seizures are controlled or adverse effects occur. If the second drug also fails in monotherapy, a combination of two drugs appropriate to the seizure type may be tried.

**consider second-line drugs**

*If the seizures remain uncontrolled, attention should again be directed to the diagnosis of epilepsy and underlying aetiology of the seizures.* One of the first-line drugs (whichever is least well-tolerated) should then gradually be replaced by a second-line drug; if the latter is effective, subsequent gradual withdrawal of the initial drug can be considered. Other second-line drugs may be tried in turn if the seizures remain intractable, and the use of experimental antiepileptic agents considered, preferably as part of a controlled trial.

### 7.9 What problems are encountered when antiepileptic drugs are used in patients with renal or hepatic disease?

**metabolism in the liver and kidney**

Sodium valproate is contraindicated in patients with active liver disease, in whom it may cause acute hepatic failure. Other antiepileptic drugs which are metabolised in the liver include carbamazepine, phenytoin, phenobarbitone, ethosuximide, lamotrigine, the benzodiazepines, and paraldehyde. These drugs should be used with caution in patients with hepatic impairment.

Drugs which are excreted via the kidney, at least in part, or which have active metabolites which are excreted in the urine include ethosuximide, phenobarbitone, the benzodiazepines, vigabatrin, lamotrigine and gabapentin, and care should be taken if these drugs are given to patients with renal impairment. Acetazolamide should be avoided if renal impairment is severe.

## 7.10 What precautions should be taken when prescribing antiepileptic drugs for the elderly?

*A special effort should be made to avoid polytherapy in the elderly, both because of the risk of drug interactions and the difficulties which may be encountered in coping with a complicated regime.*

**drug interaction in the elderly**

Compliance may be improved if instructions for taking the drugs are written down. There is an increased susceptibility to certain drugs, particularly those which may cause sedation, in old age, and such drugs should be used with care. It should also be remembered that many elderly people have a degree of renal impairment.

## 7.11 When should antiepileptic drug levels be monitored?

*The dose of drug required by each patient depends largely on the clinical response*. In general, if a patient fails to respond to a small dose of an appropriate drug, the dose should be gradually increased until either seizures are controlled, or evidence of toxicity or other adverse effects occur. However, situations in which drug-level monitoring may be helpful are shown in Table 6.

**clinical response to dosages**

**Table 6.** *Indications for monitoring of serum drug levels.*

- To check compliance in patients with refractory seizures
- To guide dosage when using drugs with difficult pharmacokinetics eg. phenytoin
- To guide dosage when using polytherapy, in patients with renal *or* hepatic disease, and in patients in whom toxicity is difficult to assess (eg. those with learning difficulties)
- To guide dosage in pregnant patients
- Controlled trials of antiepileptic drugs

<table>
<tr><td>monitoring<br>serum drug<br>levels</td><td>Monitoring of serum drug levels is most helpful in the case of phenytoin, because of its non-linear kinetics. Monitoring of carbamazepine, phenobarbitone, ethosuximide, gabapentin, lamotrigine, tiagabine, topiramate and vigabatrin levels is less helpful but may be useful in selected patients.</td></tr>
</table>

### 7.12 What factors determine the likelihood of achieving seizure control?

<table>
<tr><td>good<br>prognosis<br>for idiopathic<br>epilepsies</td><td>The likelihood of achieving seizure control is determined in part by the epilepsy syndrome and seizure type. Many of the idiopathic epilepsies have a good prognosis. Primary generalised epilepsy is usually amenable to treatment with sodium valproate provided that the drug is well tolerated. However, some syndromes, such as juvenile myoclonic epilepsy, may require long-term treatment.</td></tr>
</table>

The seizures of benign epilepsy of childhood with centrotemporal spikes almost invariably remit during the second decade, and may not require treatment at all if infrequent. Benign epilepsy of childhood with occipital paroxysms also has an excellent prognosis. In contrast, other syndromes such as West syndrome and Lennox-Gastaut syndrome imply a poor prognosis, both for seizure type and for intellectual development.

### 7.13 What are the adverse effects of medication?

<table>
<tr><td>effects of<br>medication</td><td>The adverse effects of AEDs fall into four groups: acute dose-related effects (intoxication), chronic toxic effects, idiosyncratic (allergic) effects and teratogenicity. Acute dose-related effects are similar for all the antiepileptic drugs, though they differ in degree: they include dizziness, ataxia, nystagmus, nausea, visual disturbances, headaches and drowsiness.</td></tr>
</table>

The chronic toxic effects of AEDs tend to be more subtle, often developing insidiously. They may affect many systems, producing neurological, haematological, hepatic, immunological, metabolic, endocrine, connective tissue, gastrointestinal and other changes, although such changes are often of little clinical significance. The most important of the chronic toxic effects are usually neurological, including sedation, lethargy, mental slowing, memory disturbance, depression, irritability and aggression.

*Idiosyncratic adverse effects usually develop soon after the initiation of the treatment, and may be potentially serious*. The drugs should be withdrawn if they occur. The most common is skin rash, which is occasionally severe, such as Stevens-Johnson syndrome or exfoliative dermatitis, but usually mild. Other serious but rare idiosyncratic effects are agranulocytosis or pancytopenia (described with phenytoin, carbamazepine and felbamate), pancreatitis and acute hepatic failure (reported with phenytoin, valproate, felbamate and lamotrigine).

**idiosyncratic effects**

Generalised lymphadenopathy and a lupus-like syndrome may also occur as allergic phenomena. Teratogenicity is discussed further in Chapter 9.

### 7.14 What help can be given to patients in whom medical management is unsuccessful?

As soon as it becomes clear that the seizures will not be easily controlled by medical means, and while second-line drugs are still being tried, consideration should be given to the suitability of the patient for epilepsy surgery (see Chapter 8). Appropriate investigations should be undertaken (including MRI if not already performed, and EEG monitoring to localise the site of seizure onset). *Epilepsy surgery is best carried out in specialist centres and contact should be made with one at an early stage*, since many specialists involved with epilepsy surgery prefer to carry out investigations themselves.

**specialist centres for surgery**

### 7.15 When and how should antiepileptic treatment be withdrawn?

The decision as to when to withdraw antiepileptic treatment is always difficult, particularly in adults in whom considerations such as driving and employment may be affected by a recurrence of seizures. The patient should be counselled about the risk of relapse and its possible consequences before any reduction in dose is undertaken. *It is usually advised that patients should have been seizure-free for at least two years, and preferably longer, before drug withdrawal is attempted.*

**withdrawal of drug treatment**

*Drugs should be withdrawn slowly over a period of several months*. If the patient is taking polytherapy, withdrawal of one drug should be completed before reduction of the dose of the other drug is undertaken.

**7.16 What is the risk of recurrence of seizures after stopping medication? What factors influence this?**

**factors influencing relapse**

Most studies suggest that the risk of recurrence of seizures after two years of seizure freedom following withdrawal of antiepileptic medication is about 20% in children and 40% in adults. *Factors influencing the likelihood of relapse include the duration of epilepsy prior to seizure control* (the prognosis being worse in those whose seizures were initially difficult to control), *the duration of remission* (the prognosis being better in those with long remission prior to drug withdrawal), *seizure type* (idiopathic epilepsy, except juvenile myoclonic epilepsy, usually having a better prognosis than symptomatic epilepsy), and *the presence of additional handicaps*.

The influence of the EEG on prognosis following drug withdrawal is controversial, some studies suggesting a relationship between the presence of epileptic abnormalities and the likelihood of relapse, while others do not confirm this. The association appears to be greater in children than adults.

**timescale for relapse**

The majority of *patients who relapse following drug withdrawal do so within one year*. If treatment is reinstituted, seizure control is usually regained, but difficulties may be experienced in approximately 15% of patients.

**7.17 Is there any treatment for epilepsy which does not require the use of drugs?**

**controlling severe epilepsy**

Not all people with epilepsy require treatment with antiepileptic drugs, either because they have very mild or infrequent seizures. *Although the majority of people with more severe epilepsy will require drug therapy, there may be other means by which their seizure control can be improved.*

**natural controlling techniques**

The avoidance of factors known to precipitate seizures has already been discussed. Other non-pharmacological methods for averting seizures depend on specific manoeuvres undertaken at the onset of an aura, to prevent progression of the seizure. Some people find that they may achieve this by intense concentration, others by relaxation. It may be helpful to teach patients breathing exercises to prevent hyperventilation, with its accompanying risk of facilitation of seizures, in these circumstances. Other techniques which may be helpful include intense motor activity or sensory stimulation.

A few children with intractable seizures, particularly in the context of Lennox-Gastaut syndrome and myoclonic-astatic epilepsy, may benefit from a high-fat diet, the so-called ketogenic diet. This diet is not useful in adults with epilepsy.

Vagal stimulation is a recent development in the treatment of epilepsy which is still being researched. It involves the long-term placement of an electrode to stimulate the vagal nerve, either continuously or on demand. It has been reported to be effective in a small proportion of patients with chronic partial epilepsy, but further evaluation is needed.

**the vagal nerve**

### 7.18 How should status epilepticus be treated?

*Status epilepticus is a neurological emergency, since the longer it is allowed to continue, the greater the risk of permanent cerebral damage, and the harder it becomes to control.*

**risk of cerebral damage**

Efforts should be directed at ensuring the adequacy of cardiorespiratory function, controlling the clinical and electrical manifestations of seizure activity, treating the underlying cause, and correcting metabolic imbalance occurring as a result of the status.

On the patient's arrival in hospital, an airway should be inserted and oxygen given. An intravenous cannula should be inserted, and blood taken for urea and electrolytes, blood glucose, serum calcium and magnesium, anticonvulsant levels (if a patient is known to have epilepsy), and full blood count. Arterial blood gases should be measured if clinically appropriate. Intravenous lorazepam or diazepam (the usual dose in adults being lorazepam 4 mg or diazepam 10-20 mg) should be administered by slow injection, care being taken to observe for any evidence of respiratory depression.

**oxygen and blood tests**

In most patients, seizure activity will cease with this treatment. However, there is a risk of recurrence of seizures as the serum level of the benzodiazepine drops, and a loading dose of phenytoin should therefore also be administered, the total dose being 15 mg/kg at a rate of less than 50 mg per minute. Cardiac monitoring should be carried out during the injection, and the blood pressure checked. In patients in whom status is due to antiepileptic drug withdrawal, the patient's usual medication should be re-established as soon as possible.

**monitor the heart and blood pressure**

**persistent**
**seizure activity**

In patients in whom seizure activity persists despite the initial dose of phenytoin, a further slow injection of phenytoin (5 mg/kg) should be given, repeated if necessary until a total of phenytoin 30 mg/kg has been

**secondary**
**disturbances**

administered. These patients are also likely to be developing secondary metabolic disturbances as a result of the status, including electrolyte imbalance, hypoglycaemia, dehydration, hyperpyrexia and lactic acidosis.

The acidosis, if mild, is likely to correct itself: the other abnormalities should be actively treated. Arterial blood gases should be measured, if not already done.

Other AEDs which may be administered at this time include chlormethiazole, given by infusion, rectal paraldehyde, or intravenous phenobarbitone. Any of these drugs may cause respiratory depression, and close monitoring is mandatory, so that the patient can be intubated and mechanically ventilated if necessary.

**EEG**
**monitoring**

In patients in whom all other measures fail, elective ventilation in association with thiopentone infusion may be necessary. In this instance, EEG monitoring is necessary to ensure that suppression of seizure activity is complete. EEG monitoring is also important to exclude the possibility of pseudostatus epilepticus, which is common, particularly in patients referred to tertiary centres for further treatment.

### 7.19 Which antiepileptic drugs are currently available?

The following antiepileptic drugs are currently available:

| | | | |
|---|---|---|---|
| Acetazolamide | Diazepam | Nitrazepam | Tiagabine |
| ACTH | Ethosuximide | Paraldehyde | Topiramate |
| Carbamazepine | Felbamate | Phenobarbitone | Valproate |
| Chlormethiazole | Gabapentin | Phenytoin | Vigabatrin |
| Clobazam | Lamotrigine | Piracetam | |
| Clonazepam | Lorazepam | Primidone | |

### Acetazolamide

This is a sulphonamide and carbonic anhydrase inhibitor which is a second-line antiepileptic drug effective in the treatment of generalised tonic clonic, absence and complex partial seizures.

Acetazolamide's major drawback is that, in the majority of patients, tolerance develops after several months. Adverse effects include paraesthesias, malaise, anorexia and weight loss, mild diuresis, depression, lethargy and dizziness. Renal calculi may also occur, and blood dyscrasias have been reported rarely. Teratogenicity has been noted in animals.

## Adrenocorticotrophic hormone (ACTH)

This drug is said to be useful in the treatment of infantile spasms. It is given by intramuscular injection, usually in reducing doses over a period of three months.

Adverse effects of the drug include leukocytosis, irritability, hypertension, vomiting, peripheral oedema, Cushiongoid facies, gastrointestinal haemorrhage, electrolyte disturbances, reversible cerebral atrophy, sepsis, hyperglycaemia, and congestive cardiac failure.

## Carbamazepine

Carbamazepine is a tricyclic iminostilbene derivative used in the treatment of epilepsy since the 1960s, and is a first-line drug in the treatment of generalised tonic clonic, simple partial and complex partial seizures. It may exacerbate generalised absence seizures.

Carbamazepine is available in tablet form, suppositories, and liquid, but not as an injectable preparation. It is metabolised in the liver, and causes induction of hepatic enzymes, so that the metabolism of drugs such as oral contraceptive agents and warfarin is increased.

The usual daily dose of carbamazepine in adults is 400-1800 mg. Toxic symptoms are common if the dose of the drug is increased quickly, and may also occur during long term administration as a time-locked phenomenon after each dose. The symptoms in the latter situation may be ameliorated by taking a smaller dose more frequently, or through the use of controlled-release preparations of carbamazepine.

The most common unwanted effect of carbamazepine is skin rash, which occurs in up to 10% of patients and may be serious in up to 5%. Other adverse effects include nausea, diplopia, nystagmus, dizziness, fatigue, and headache. Weight gain may occur, as may water retention. A mild leukopenia, usually not clinically significant, occurs in about 10% of patients. Serious idiosyncratic reactions such as agranulocytosis are rare and not easily predictable by monitoring.

### Chlormethiazole

Chlormethiazole is available as an intravenous preparation for infusion in the treatment of status epilepticus. Adverse effects include respiratory depression, tachycardia, hypotension, depressed conscious level, hyponatraemia, nasal congestion, and headache.

### Clobazam

Clobazam is a 1.5 benzodiazepine used as a second-line drug and effective against all seizure types. It is given orally, the usual dose being 10-30 mg at night to avoid daytime sedation.

As with the other benzodiazepines, tolerance occurs frequently, and has been reported in 77% of patients within eight months. In some patients however, it remains useful. Intermittent clobazam may be helpful in the management of catamenial epilepsy and taken as required in patients in whom seizures occur in clusters.

### Clonazepam

Clonazepam is particularly helpful in the treatment of myoclonus and photosensitive seizures, although it may also be beneficial as a second-line drug in most seizure types. It is useful in the generalised epilepsies in patients unable to tolerate valproate. The starting dose is 0.5 mg, increasing if necessary to a total dose of up to 8 mg.

Clonazepam is also available as an intravenous preparation for infusion in the treatment of status epilepticus. Sedation is more common than with clobazam, occurring initially in up to 50% of patients, although this symptom often improves with time. Other adverse effects include ataxia, muscle weakness, behaviour problems, nausea, hypersalivation, weight gain, and rarely, haematological effects.

Tolerance is less common than with clobazam, developing in about 30% of patients. The drug should be withdrawn slowly to avoid the risk of withdrawal seizures.

**Diazepam**

This drug is used in the management of serial seizures and status epilepticus. There is no place for it in the maintenance treatment of epilepsy. It is usually given intravenously in the treatment of status epilepticus, the typical dose in adults being 10-20 mg. Its use in this situation is to some extent superseded by the use of intravenous lorazepam.

Seizures may recur as the plasma level falls, and therefore the administration of additional medication (such as intravenous phenytoin) is advisable in addition. Diazepam is also rapidly absorbed rectally and this is a useful route of administration in the treatment of serial or prolonged seizures, allowing administration by parents or other carers and potentially avoiding the need for hospital admission.

Adverse effects include sedation, respiratory depression, hypotension, obtundation, drowsiness, vertigo, ataxia, blurred vision and amnesia.

**Ethosuximide**

The only use of ethosuximide is in the treatment of true absence (petit mal) seizures; where these co-exist with other seizure types, valproate is usually the first treatment of choice. Ethosuximide is available in tablet form and syrup, the usual starting dose being 250 mg, increased to a typical maintenance dose of 15-20 mg/kg/day.

Drug level monitoring may be helpful. Adverse effects include nausea and vomiting, anorexia, abdominal discomfort, sedation, psychoses, movement disorders, and skin rash. Serious hypersensitivity reactions occur rarely. Valproate decreases the clearance of ethosuximide and may cause toxicity.

**Felbamate**

Felbamate is a di-carbamate closely related to meprobamate and may be used as a drug of last resort in patients with intractable epilepsy, particularly the Lennox-Gastaut syndrome. Its exact mechanism of action is not known but it appears to prevent seizure spread by both increasing seizure threshold and acting on voltage-dependent sodium channels. It is available in 400 and 600 mg tablets. The usual dose is between 1,200 and 3,600 mg/day. Felbamate exhibits significant pharmacokinetic interactions with phenytoin, carbamazepine and valproic acid. Plasma phenytoin concentrations rise by 20% in patients upon introduction of felbamate. Plasma carbamazepine concentrations are reduced by 20-25% upon felbamate co-administration. This has been associated with concurrent increases in carbamazepine epoxide concentrations.

In patients taking valproic acid, plasma valproic acid concentrations have been elevated by approximately 50% during comedication with felbamate. The exact mechanism of these interactions is unknown but their magnitude suggests that dosage adjustments will be necessary if seizure control is to be maintained and side-effects are to be avoided during polytherapy. Felbamate metabolism is also inducible by carbamazepine and phenytoin, and thus higher felbamate doses will be necessary during co-administration with these antiepileptic drugs.

The most frequently reported side effects during felbamate therapy have been neurological (diplopia, insomnia, dizziness, headache and ataxia), and gastrointestinal (anorexia, nausea and vomiting). A major use-limiting problem is its potential to cause aplastic anaemia and liver failure, affecting as many as one in 4,000 patients exposed to the drug. Hence, it seems prudent to limit its use to specialist centres in severe intractable cases.

**Gabapentin**

Gabapentin is a chemical derivative of GABA and was originally designed to mimic the action of GABA in the brain. Subsequent studies, however, have shown that gabapentin is inactive at GABA receptors.

More recent studies have shown that gabapentin interacts with a specific high affinity binding site in the brain that has as yet not been identified. It appears, however, to be associated with a leucine transporter system across neuronal cell membranes. Gabapentin may increase intracellular concentration of GABA by modulating leucine transport across cell membranes and increasing the activity of glutamic acid decarboxylase. If this proves true, then gabapentin is the first drug of a new family of antiepileptic drugs in terms of its mechanism of action.

Gabapentin is used as second line treatment of partial seizures, with or without secondary generalisation in patients not controlled by or intolerant to other antiepileptic drugs. The optimal dose remains to be established but the maximum recommended dose is currently 2400 mg/day. The efficacy of higher doses is presently being investigated in clinical trials.

The recommended initial dose of gabapentin is 300-400 mg/day, and the suggested titration rate consists of daily dose increases up to 900-1200 mg/day in the first instance. Many experienced clinicians, however, recommend a much slower rate with weekly incremental steps rather than a daily basis. In view of its pharmacokinetic profile, a three times daily dosage is recommended, but many patients are able to use a twice daily regimen without any problems.

The efficacy of gabapentin has been shown in three large controlled trials. Data from these studies suggest a significant seizure decrease in up to a quarter of patients exposed to it.

Gabapentin has a very desirable pharmacokinetic profile as it is not metabolised, exhibits no protein binding and does not induce hepatic enzymes. Its potential for drug interactions is, therefore, small, and to date no clinically significant interactions with other AEDs or other drugs have been reported. There is no need to measure its plasma concentration as a guide to dosing.

Gabapentin is usually well tolerated and its side effects are mainly related to the CNS. The most frequently reported side effect is drowsiness; others include dizziness, diplopia, ataxia and headache. Gabapentin treatment has not been associated with any serious idiosyncratic reaction. It may be a useful add-on drug in patients with a high risk of drug interactions such as the elderly, and in children with learning difficulties where cognitive functions are an important consideration.

### Lamotrigine

Lamotrigine was originally developed for its antifolate activity following suggestions of a relationship between folates and epilepsy. Its mode of action, however, is not related to its weak antifolate property and is now thought to be due mainly to its potential to modulate sodium channels and to block the pathological release of glutamate, an important substrate for excitatory transmission.

Lamotrigine was first licensed as a second line drug for refractory epilepsy. Recently, the terms of its licence have been extended to cover use as a first line drug in patients with partial seizures, with or without secondary generalisation, and in generalised tonic clonic convulsions.

The recommended starting dose is 25 mg when used in monotherapy. When used as add-on therapy, the initial dose is 25 mg given on alternate days in patients receiving concomitant sodium valproate with a usual maximum of 100-200 mg daily and 50 mg daily in patients receiving other AEDs, with a maximum recommended dose of 400 mg/day in two divided doses.

Treatment should be slowly titrated upwards over a period of several weeks. Too rapid titration may be associated with an increased incidence of adverse events particularly skin rash.

The efficacy of lamotrigine as an antiepileptic drug has been evaluated in several controlled studies in patients with mainly partial seizures. The pooled data of these studies has shown that 22% of patients have more than a 50% reduction in seizure frequency, but only a few become seizure free.

A recent comparative study between lamotrigine and carbamazepine in newly diagnosed epilepsy suggests that both drugs have similar efficacy. There have been many anecdotal reports of a higher efficacy of lamotrigine in patients with idiopathic generalised epilepsies but this has not yet been formally tested.

Lamotrigine does not appear to interact with other concomitantly administered antiepileptic drugs. Hepatic enzyme inducers, however, boost the metabolism of lamotrigine reducing its half life. Higher doses of lamotrigine need to be administered therefore, if it is used in conjunction with enzyme inducing drugs such as phenytoin and carbamazepine.

On the other hand, inhibitors of hepatic enzymes such as sodium valproate block the metabolism of lamotrigine, and reduced doses of lamotrigine need to be used if these drugs are given in combination.

Headaches, drowsiness, ataxia and diplopia (usually transient) are the most commonly reported acute adverse effects, particularly during dose escalation. Skin rash is the most common idiosyncratic side effect of this drug and affects up to 8-10% of patients. A much higher incidence was observed during early studies when larger initial doses of lamotrigine than presently recommended were used. There have been a few reports of fatalities due to disseminated intravascular coagulation and fulminant liver failure associated with the use of lamotrigine. These rare events, however, have to be seen in the context of more than 100,000 patients exposed to the drug.

## Lorazepam

Lorazepam, given intravenously, controls seizures in 80-90% of patients with status epilepticus. In adults, it is given in a dose of 4 mg over 2 minutes, repeated if necessary after 15 minutes. Adverse effects include sedation, amnesia, dysarthria, delirium, hallucinations, and respiratory depression.

## Nitrazepam

Nitrazepam is used in the treatment of infantile spasms, and has been shown to have a similar efficacy to that of ACTH. As with other benzodiazepines, tolerance may occur.

## Paraldehyde

This drug may be helpful in the treatment of serial seizures and status epilepticus. It is usually given rectally; if a plastic syringe is used the drug must be given immediately since it reacts with plastics.

## Phenobarbitone

Phenobarbitone has been used in the treatment of epilepsy since 1912 and remains a useful adjunct in the treatment of generalised tonic clonic and partial seizures in patients not responding to, or intolerant of, other drugs. Its adverse effects include sedation and behavioural problems in children, and as a result it is now not usually used as a first-line drug. Other effects include reduction of serum and red cell folate, disorders of calcium metabolism, connective tissue disorders such as Dupuytren's contracture, and depression. Serious idiosyncratic reactions occur rarely.

The mode of action of phenobarbitone is probably mediated by the GABA receptor, though it is not clearly defined. The drug is largely metabolised in the liver, and as in the case of phenytoin and carbamazepine, induction of hepatic enzymes occurs.

**Phenytoin**

Phenytoin is an effective drug in the treatment of tonic-clonic, tonic, and partial seizures, and may also be helpful in the treatment of atonic seizures and atypical absences. It is not helpful in typical generalised absences (which it may exacerbate) and myoclonic seizures. Tolerance to its antiepileptic action does not usually occur.

Phenytoin is available as capsules, tablets, suspension and injection. There may be differences in bioavailability between the different oral preparations and patients stabilised on one formulation should continue to receive the same formulation.

The usual daily dose, which may be given as a single dose, is 250-400 mg. Intravenous phenytoin is useful in patients unable to take the drug by the gastroinstestinal route, and those with serial seizures or in status epilepticus. Since it may cause heart block it should be administered with caution and at a rate not exceeding 50 mg/minute. It should never be given intramuscularly, since absorption by this route is slow and unreliable, and tissue necrosis may occur.

Phenytoin has non-linear kinetics and a low therapeutic index and in some patients frequent drug serum level measurements may be necessary as a guide to dosing. Drug interactions are common as phenytoin metabolism is very susceptible to inhibition by certain drugs, and it may enhance the metabolism of other drugs. Caution should therefore be exercised when other medications are introduced or withdrawn.

Adverse effects are common, occurring in up to half of patients treated with phenytoin, although drug withdrawal is necessary in only about 10%, most commonly due to skin rash. Dose related adverse reactions including nystagmus, ataxia, and lethargy are common.

Cosmetic effects such as gum hypertrophy, hirsutism, and acne are well-recognised adverse effects and should be taken into account when prescribing for children and young women. Chronic adverse effects include folate deficiency, osteomalacia, Dupuytren's contractures and cerebellar atrophy. Serious idiosyncratic adverse events, including hepatic failure and bone marrow depression are extremely uncommon.

**Piracetam**

Piracetam is a pyrrolidine acetamate that has been used as a memory "enhancer" in some European countries for a number of years; it has, however, never been shown to be effective. Recently, it was found that piracetam is a very effective anti-myoclonic drug. The mode of action of this drug is unknown.

Piracetam is available in tablets of 800 mg and also in oral solution of 333 mg/ml. The usual dose ranges from 7,200 mg to 20,000 mg. There is no known drug interaction and it has relatively few side effects. Diarrhoea, weight gain, insomnia, depression and hyperkinesia have been associated with it, particularly in high doses.

**Primidone**

Primidone is metabolised to phenobarbitone and phenylethylmalonamide, and there has been controversy as to whether it has any antiepileptic effect over and above that of phenobarbitone itself. Any such effect appears to be slight.

In one study comparing phenobarbitone with primidone in patients with partial and secondarily generalised seizures, the efficacy of the two drugs was similar but primidone caused significantly more adverse effects. Acute toxicity, causing dizziness, weakness, drowsiness and ataxia may occur following the first dose. This is minimised by starting the drug at a low dose (eg 125 mg) taken at night. Other adverse effects are similar to those of phenobarbitone.

**Tiagabine**

Tiagabine is a specific inhibitor of gamma-aminobutyric acid (GABA) uptake in glial cells and nerve terminals. Uptake inhibition leads to a rise in extracellular GABA and consequently increases GABA neurotransmission. Tiagabine is effective in a wide range of animal seizure models, predictive of a broad spectrum of antiepileptic activity.

Tiagabine is rapidly absorbed after oral ingestion, reaching peak concentration within one hour. Food reduces the rate, but not the extent of absorption and thus the timing of a dose in relation to meals is unlikely to be clinically relevant. Tiagabine exhibits linear kinetics. Elimination half-life in healthy volunteers is 5-13 hours and is not dose-dependent, but it may be reduced to 2-3 hours in patients on concomitant enzyme inducing antiepileptic drugs. Despite this short half-life, three doses per days have been found to be therapeutically effective. Tiagabine does not affect the levels of carbamazepine or phenytoin, but may reduce the plasma concentration of valproate by about 10% (this is unlikely to be clinically important). Tiagabine has not been shown to interact with the contraceptive pill.

Tiagabine has been shown to be an effective antiepileptic drug against partial seizures with or without secondary generalisation in five placebo controlled trials in which a dose response effect was observed. In these patients with epilepsy not sufficiently controlled with currently available antiepileptic drugs, for instance, tiagabine reduced complex partial seizures by at least 50% in 27% of patients but this was increased to 42% when the analysis was restricted to those in the higher dose groups.

In clinical trials tiagabine's main side effects were transient, usually mild to moderate, primarily central nervous system related and occurred mostly during drug titration; the main side effects being sedation, headache, tiredness and dizziness. Tremor, diarrhoea and depressed mood also occurred statistically more frequently in those taking tiagabine compared with those taking placebo. The safety of tiagabine has been confirmed in open label studies with a total exposure of over 2,100 patients (this number would be able to detect with 95% confidence a serious adverse event that occurred with an incidence of about 1 in 700 patients).

As add-on therapy, tiagabine should be started at 7.5-15 mg/day in 3 divided doses, and increased by 5-15 mg/day each week up to the minimum effective dose, which is usually 30 mg/day. The maximum recommended dose is 50 mg/day, although higher doses (up to 70 mg/day) have been well-tolerated. No dosage adjustments are necessary in children (>12 years), the elderly and in patients with renal impairment.

**Topiramate**

Topiramate is chemically unrelated to other AEDs, and to date four possible mechanisms of action have been identified to account for its mode of action. It is a strong blocker of voltage-activated sodium channels and has a marked effect on GABA-A receptors. In addition, it blocks the kainate/AMPA type of glutamate receptors and is a weak inhibitor of carbonic anhydrase. It is not clear if this is relevant to its antiepileptic action.

Topiramate is used as a second line drug for patients with partial seizures with or without secondary generalisation who are inadequately controlled on first line antiepileptic drugs. Recommended doses are between 200-600 mg although some patients may derive benefit in doses that are outside this range.

The recommended starting dose for most patients is 50 mg once daily, titrating upwards in 50 mg/day increments at weekly intervals up to 200 mg/day in two divided doses. After that, the dose should be increased by 100 mg each week until seizure control is achieved or side effects develop.

Topiramate efficacy was assessed in five controlled trials in patients with partial seizures. There was a 50% reduction of seizure frequency in 48% of patients. Anecdotal reports of its efficacy in other seizure types, particularly in idiopathic generalised epilepsy and in Lennox-Gastaut, need to be formally confirmed.

Topiramate exhibits linear pharmacokinetics with low levels of protein binding. It has minimal interaction with other AEDs, although hepatic enzyme inducers accelerate its metabolism. Because of this, topiramate doses may need to be adjusted downwards if patients are coming off carbamazepine or phenytoin. Topiramate also has the potential to interact with the oral contraceptive pill and it is advisable that women taking topiramate use one with an increased oestrogen content.

Most acute and dose related side effects of topiramate are CNS-related. These include dizziness, drowsiness, nervousness, impaired concentration, and fatigue. They are mostly transient and related to dose and rate of titration. Parasthesias and nephrolithiasis ~ 1.5% have also been reported and are likely to be due to topiramate's carbonic anhydrase inhibitory action. Patients starting topiramate should increase their fluid intake to reduce the risk of kidney stones reported up to 1.5 years after discontinuation of treatment. Weight loss is seen in up to 20% of patients. Topiramate has been shown to be teratogenic in some animal models and should be used with caution in women of child-bearing age.

**Valproate**

This is a branched chain fatty acid which is usually prescribed as the sodium salt in Europe. It is very effective in the treatment of the primary generalised epilepsies, and also in the treatment of secondarily generalised seizures. Its precise mode of action is unknown, although it may be in part due to an increase in brain GABA levels.

Valproate is available orally in tablet, syrup and liquid form, and is also made as an intravenous preparation for patients temporarily unable to take the drug orally (its onset of action is not rapid enough for it to be useful in the treatment of status epilepticus).

The usual daily maintenance dose in adults ranges from 600-2500 mg. It is almost entirely metabolised in the liver, and its metabolism is thus affected by such drugs as carbamazepine and phenytoin. Sodium valproate itself does not induce liver enzymes.

The most serious adverse effect of valproate is hepatotoxicity, which may be fatal. This usually occurs in very young children within 3 months of starting medication, particularly in those with mental retardation and those on polytherapy for their epilepsy, and is generally heralded by abdominal pain, nausea and lethargy. Pancreatitis may also occur in patients taking valproate.

Other adverse effects include nausea and vomiting, weight gain, hair loss, and tremor, which may be dose-related. About 40% of patients taking valproate experience a benign increase in liver enzymes. Stupor, coma and reversible dementia have rarely been reported. Inhibition of platelet aggregation occurs but is not usually a problem except after surgery.

**Vigabatrin**

Vigabatrin is an irreversible inhibitor of GABA-aminotransferase, the effect of which is to increase GABA levels in the CSF by up to 150% within days of starting treatment.

Vigabatrin is indicated for use as a second line treatment for patients with partial seizures with or without secondary generalisation, and is the drug of choice for infantile spasms. The recommended dose in adults is 1000-2000 mg/day, although doses of up to 4000 mg/day in two divided doses can be used if necessary.

Contrary to initial recommendations, treatment should be started with a low dose (250-500 mg/day), and titrated slowly upwards over a period of several weeks until therapeutic response is achieved. Too rapid titration may be associated with an increased incidence of adverse events.

The efficacy of vigabatrin as an antiepileptic drug has been extensively demonstrated in a number of studies. Overall, these studies have shown that 40-50% of patients with refractory partial seizures have more than a 50% reduction in seizure frequency. In general the greatest efficacy has been noted against complex partial seizures.

There is little data on efficacy against primary generalised epilepsy and it may worsen myoclonic seizures. There is, however, good evidence for the use of vigabatrin in infantile spasms. Long term follow-up studies have shown that an initial good response is maintained in over 60% of patients but tolerance may develop in up to a third of patients.

The addition of vigabatrin results in a fall in the plasma concentrations of phenytoin by an average of 25%. The mechanism for this is not established but it may be due to decreased phenytoin absorption. In most patients this has no clinical significance, but occasionally an increase in phenytoin dose is necessary if there is an increase in seizures a few weeks after the introduction of vigabatrin.

The corollary of this effect is that plasma phenytoin concentrations rise by an average of 25% after the withdrawal of concomitant vigabatrin therapy. Vigabatrin has virtually no phamacokinetic interactions with other antiepileptic drugs. There is no need to measure the plasma concentration to guide dosing.

Sedation, dizziness and headache are the most commonly reported acute adverse effects, particularly when doses are being increased. Tolerance often develops so that the symptoms are frequently self-limiting. These symptoms can usually be avoided by introducing the drug gradually. Allergic skin rashes are extremely rare.

Up to 10% of patients taking vigabatrin develop changes in mood. Most common are agitation, ill temper and disturbed behaviour, or depression. Overall, up to 4% of patients on vigabatrin may develop paranoid and psychotic symptoms. The incidence of severe psychiatric and behavioural adverse effects appears to have reduced recently, probably because of the trend towards slower introduction of the drug and awareness of the initial symptoms of psychiatric disturbance that may resolve on dose reduction. In clinical practice it is important to warn patients and carers of possible adverse effects, and to give advice on tapering the medication should these occur.

# CHAPTER 8

## THE SURGICAL TREATMENT OF EPILEPSY

### 8.1 When should surgical treatment be considered for epilepsy?

In some patients epilepsy is a symptom of a pathological process which can be identified by CT or MRI scanning, while in others the nature of the underlying cause remains unknown despite investigation with currently available technology. In either instance, the seizures may be amenable to treatment by surgical means. If the underlying lesion is progressive (such as a tumour) or carries other inherent risks (such as the risk of haemorrhage from an arteriovenous malformation) the need for surgery may be determined by these considerations, regardless of seizure frequency. In patients without such a lesion, other criteria must be used to determine whether epilepsy surgery is appropriate.

The criteria for treating epilepsy by surgical means vary somewhat from centre to centre. There is wide agreement that *epilepsy should have been shown to be intractable to medical treatment before surgery is contemplated*. Such a trial of therapy should include treatment with at least two first-line drugs appropriate to the type of epilepsy separately, and with adequate compliance. Although it is often reasonable to try several different drugs alone or together over a period of time, the chance of a patient becoming seizure-free diminishes if control is not achieved with initial first-line drugs, and evaluation for surgery should not be unduly delayed while every possible combination of medication is tried.

*medication vs surgery*

*Epilepsy surgery is a major undertaking, and is usually only considered in patients with frequent seizures*. Some centres suggest as a minimum an average of at least one seizure per week, but others consider patients with less frequent attacks, if they are severe enough to significantly interfere with life style. Because of the physical and emotional strains of preoperative evaluation as well as the surgery itself, all patients should undergo psychological and psychiatric assessment, and only those patients with the resources to cope, either with surgery or the fact that surgery may not be helpful, should be offered further evaluation.

*sugery is a major undertaking*

**IQ may determine suitability for surgery**

*Some surgeons consider that a low IQ is a contraindication to epilepsy surgery since it reflects diffuse brain damage, and clinicians may not contemplate preoperative evaluation in patients with an IQ of less than 70.* However, patients with a lower IQ may derive benefit, for example by the abolition by corpus callosotomy of frequent tonic or atonic attacks causing injury, and should therefore receive consideration of operative measures if appropriate.

### 8.2 What types of surgical treatment are available?

**removing the epileptic focus**

There are two main strategies for the surgical treatment of seizures. The first involves resective surgery, in which the aim of the *surgery is the removal of the epileptic focus itself*. Examples of this type of surgery are anterior temporal lobectomy (Figure 21), selective amygdalo-hippocampectomy (in which only the mesial temporal structures are removed), or resection of a frontal lobe lesion. At the other extreme of resective surgery, in patients in whom most or all of one hemisphere is abnormal, as in hemimegalencephaly or Rasmussen's encephalitis (an uncommon inflammatory condition causing seizures, progressive hemiparesis and intellectual deterioration), hemispherectomy may be necessary. The other strategy for surgical treatment is to interrupt the pathways of seizure spread, thus isolating the epileptic focus from the rest

**isolating the epileptic focus**

of the brain to a greater or lesser extent. Examples of this type of surgery include section of the corpus callosum, and multiple subpial transection. Callosotomy was devised to prevent secondary generalisation of seizures, and its chief indication is in the treatment of intractable generalised seizures, particularly atonic seizures.

The procedure is sometimes carried out in two stages to try to avoid disconnection syndromes, in the hope that anterior callosotomy may provide satisfactory seizure control without the need for further surgery. Multiple subpial transection is a technique which relies on the fact that seizure spread in general occurs in a tangential manner through the cerebral cortex, while impulses controlling voluntary movement travel radially. In this operation, multiple cuts are made vertically in the cortex in an effort to isolate the epileptogenic area from the surrounding cortex. It may be helpful in the treatment of seizures arising in eloquent areas of the brain, such as the speech area or motor cortex.

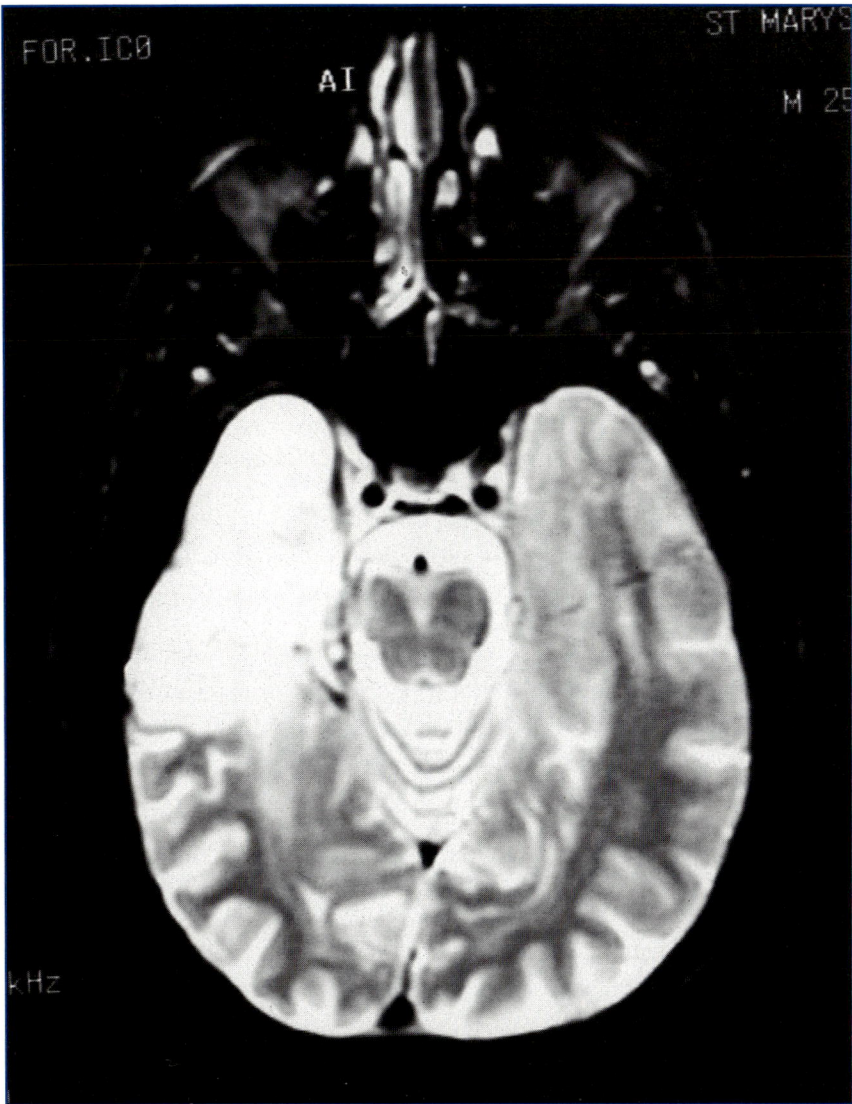

**Figure 21.** *MRI scan showing anterior temporal lobe resection.*
*(Courtesy of Dr Sanjay Sisodiya).*

### 8.3 What determines the type and extent of surgery?

*The type of surgery is dependent on the underlying lesion, its site and extent.* The most common type of surgery undertaken for epilepsy is temporal lobe surgery, either anterior temporal resection (Figure 21), or selective amygdalohippocampectomy which has superseded the more extensive surgery in a number of centres in recent years. Frontal lobe

surgery is
dependent on
the lesion site
and extent

resection is carried out less commonly, and resection of the other lobes less often still, usually if a radiological lesion is present. Hemispherectomy is indicated in patients with infantile hemiplegia (or hemiplegia developing in childhood as a result of chronic encephalitis) and seizures arising from the diseased hemisphere.

In general, patients with multifocal or generalised epilepsy are not suitable for epilepsy surgery, except possibly corpus callosotomy. Until recently, patients in whom the epileptic focus was situated in a functionally eloquent area were also considered unsuitable: however, multiple subpial transection may occasionally be helpful in such cases.

### 8.4 What evaluation is necessary prior to carrying out surgery?

**evaluation of the epileptic focus**

*Pre-operative evaluation is largely directed towards the precise localisation of the epileptic focus, and the need to ensure that resection will not compromise cognitive functions such as memory and speech.*

**maintaining cognitive functions**

Initial, non-invasive investigation includes interictal EEG studies during wakefulness and sleep, usually with sphenoidal or other electrodes suitable for recording from the anterior temporal region, neuroimaging (CT and/or MRI scan, including volumetric assessment of the mesial temporal structures where appropriate), and neuropsychological and psychiatric

**non-invasive investigations**

assessment. If a structural lesion is identified radiologically and is concordant with the seizure pattern, EEG findings (both epileptic activity and background abnormalities), and neuropsychological findings, surgery may be possible without further investigation. If these conditions do not prevail, further investigation may be required, including prolonged EEG video monitoring, with reduction of antiepileptic drugs if necessary, to obtain an ictal EEG. A Wada test, in which sodium amytal is injected

**invasive investigations**

into each carotid artery in turn and tests of speech and memory carried out, may be necessary to lateralise cognitive function and predict any post-operative deficits.

If the site of seizure onset remains uncertain after these investigations, for example if there is discordance between the clinical seizure pattern and epileptic focus, or the apparent epileptic focus does not correspond to neuroradiological abnormalities, more invasive investigation with intracranial electrodes (such as depth electrodes or subdural electrodes) may be indicated. Further information as to the probable site of seizure onset may be obtained from functional imaging with SPECT or PET scans.

## 8.5 How effective is surgery in the treatment of epilepsy?

The outcome of epilepsy surgery may be examined either in terms of seizure control alone, or with respect to its effect on wider issues, including psychiatric and social functioning.

**Table 7.** *Classification of outcome after epilepsy surgery.*

---

### Class I: Seizure-free (excluding early post-operative seizures)
**A** Completely seizure-free since surgery
**B** Aura only since surgery
**C** Some seizures after surgery, but seizure-free for at least 2 years
**D** Atypical generalised convulsion with antiepileptic drug withdrawal only

### Class II: Rare seizures ("almost seizure-free")
**A** Initially seizure-free but rare seizures now
B Rare seizures since surgery
**C** More than rare seizures after surgery, but rare seizures for at least 2 years
**D** Nocturnal seizures only, which cause no disability

### Class III: Worthwhile improvement
**A** Worthwhile seizure reduction
**B** Prolonged seizure-free intervals amounting to greater than half the follow-up period, but not less than 2 years

### Class IV: No worthwhile improvement
**A** Significant seizure reduction
**B** No appreciable change
**C** Seizures worse

(Engel J. (ed) Surgical Treatment of Epilepsy. New York: Raven Press 1993).

---

*Seizures occurring in the immediate postoperative period are not necessarily predictive of long-term outcome*, and are often excluded from the assessment of post-operative seizure control. Following surgery, many patients remain entirely seizure-free. Some patients continue to have seizures, but at a decreasing frequency, and their seizures may eventually "run down" and stop over a period of months or years. Still others are seizure-free immediately after surgery, and for months or years thereafter, when a recurrence of their attacks occurs. Auras may continue to occur after surgery in some people, and if they do not progress to other seizures

*predicting long-term outcome*

or interfere with daily life, such patients are usually considered to be "seizure-free".  Based on these considerations, a classification of outcome following surgery has been devised by Engel (Table 7).

**freedom from seizures**
The overall outcome with respect to seizure freedom depends on many factors, including the selection of patients for surgery, the underlying pathology (Figure 22), the length of follow-up, the centre carrying out the surgery, and the policy regarding antiepileptic medication after surgery. It is common experience in reputable centres that at least 60% of patients become seizure-free after anterior temporal lobectomy, 45% after extratemporal resection, 75% after hemispherectomy, and 5% after corpus callosotomy (although a much larger percentage show some improvement).

**psychosocial outcome**
With regard to psychosocial outcome after epilepsy surgery, a number of studies have shown some improvement in the majority of patients.  The areas addressed in these studies have included interpersonal relationships, vocational adjustment, dependence, personal adjustment, and overall psychosocial functioning.  However, such improvements are often limited to those patients becoming seizure-free or almost so.  Even among patients experiencing good control of their seizures following surgery, a favourable psychosocial outcome is not guaranteed and an increased suicide rate has been reported after epilepsy surgery both in patients with a good and those with a poor result.

### 8.6 What are the risks of epilepsy surgery?

**the risks of surgical complications**
The hazards of epileptic surgery embrace both the hazards of any neurosurgical procedure, and the specific hazards of the operation. Among the general risks of neurosurgery are those of death, haemorrhage, and infection.  The complications of temporal lobectomy include the possibility of hemiparesis (possibly due to manipulation of the middle cerebral artery), dysphasia, visual field defects, and damage to memory functions.

*The risk of operative complications varies from centre to centre depending on the degree of experience and technical expertise of the surgeon*.  The overall mortality of temporal lobectomy is less than 0.5%, and the risk of permanent hemiparesis less than 1%.  However, a quadrantic field defect is usual.  This is not the case with selective amygdalo-hippocampectomy.  Frontal lobe resection also carries a risk of motor and sensory defects and speech deficits.

In the past, classical (anatomic) hemispherectomies were complicated in as many as one third of instances by the development of superficial cerebral haemosiderosis, causing obstructive hydrocephalus and progressive neurological deficits. Such complications have been largely prevented by the development of the procedures of modified hemispherectomy and functional hemispherectomy. In the former, the volume of the hemispheric cavity is reduced by sewing the dural flap to the falx and tentorium, thus creating a large extradural space. In a functional hemispherectomy, large parts of the frontal and occipital regions are left in situ, but disconnected from the rest of the brain. Mutism, akinesis and occasionally hemiparesis may be seen after corpus callosotomy, but are usually transient. Disconnection syndromes sometimes develop, particularly if a complete callosotomy is performed. Psychiatric complications may also occur, following epilepsy surgery and an increased incidence of suicide has been reported even in patients becoming seizure-free.

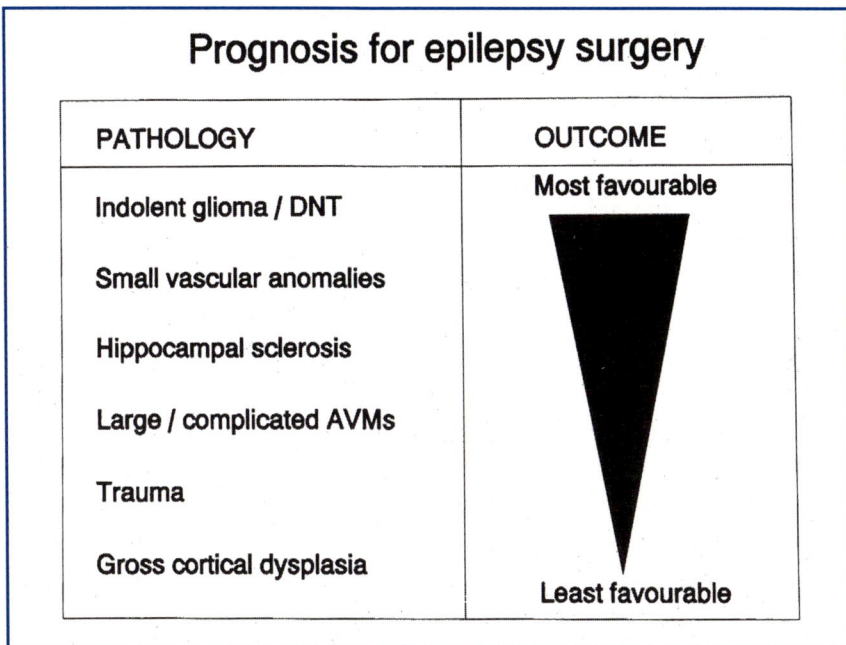

**modified and functional hemispherec-tomies**

**Figure 22.** *Diagram to show prognosis following epilepsy surgery according to aetiology. Reproduced with permission from: Duncan JS, Fish DR, Shorvon SD. Clinical Epilepsy. Edinburgh, Churchill Livingstone, 1995.*

# CHAPTER 9

## EPILEPSY IN WOMEN

**9.1 Can seizures occurring in association with menstruation be helped by hormonal treatment?**

Approximately two thirds of women with epilepsy complain of an increase in seizures at the time of menstruation, but the term *catamenial epilepsy should technically be reserved for those patients whose seizures only occur immediately preceding or during menstruation* - probably about 5% of women with epilepsy. Several possible mechanisms have been put forward for this increase in seizure frequency, including the increase in the oestrogen:progesterone ratio which occurs at this time, fluid and electrolyte imbalance, a fall in the level of antiepileptic drugs, and increased stress as a result of premenstrual tension.

**menstruation and seizures**

Various hormonal and other treatments have been used for catamenial epilepsy. Unfortunately they have been tried mostly in individual or small groups of patients (often those with intractable epilepsy which is not strictly catamenial) in an open-label, add-on manner, and the success of these manoeuvres is thus difficult to judge, although it appears to be limited. Progesterone has been reported to cause a decrease in seizures in some women. Oestrogens, on the other hand, have been shown to cause an increased susceptibility to seizures in animal models. Clomiphene has been used in selected women with anovulatory cycles or inadequate luteal phases on the basis that reportedly seizure frequency had been increased in these women, and this treatment produced some improvement in the majority. However, the evidence that the treatment significantly improves catamenial epilepsy is slight. The effect of diuretics appears to be similarly limited. Intermittent treatment with adjunctive second-line antiepileptic drugs, such as acetazolamide or clobazam has been advocated, and appears to help in some women.

**the effects of hormones as treatment**

**9.2** **What advice should be given to people with epilepsy regarding contraception?**

**decreased efficacy of oral contraceptives**

Those antiepileptic drugs (carbamazepine, phenytoin, phenobarbitone, primidone and tiagabine) which cause induction of hepatic enzymes are associated with a decreased efficacy of oral contraceptive agents, presumably as a result of increased hepatic metabolism of these agents. This may often be overcome by using a contraceptive pill with an increased oestrogen content. If breakthrough bleeding occurs, this should be taken as an indication that the agent may not provide adequate contraception, and a barrier method used in addition for the rest of the cycle. However, the absence of breakthrough bleeding does not guarantee the efficacy of the oral contraceptive pill. Women taking topiramate should also use a contraceptive pill with an increased oestrogen content.

**9.3** **What effect does epilepsy have on fertility?**

**epilepsy's effect on fertility**

Studies suggest that fertility in women with epilepsy is decreased compared to the general population, although the reasons for this are complex. It has been reported that people with epilepsy are more likely to remain single than the general population, particularly if seizures develop early in life. The number of children born to married women is also lower than expected. Several studies have reported a reduction in sexual interest and activity in patients with epilepsy, particularly those with temporal lobe epilepsy.

It is likely that hormonal, social and other factors contribute to this decrease in fertility. The synthesis of sex hormone-binding globulin, which binds to testosterone and oestrogen, is increased by phenytoin, carbamazepine and phenobarbitone, thus reducing the concentration of free sex steroids. Enzyme induction by antiepileptic drugs may increase clearance of sex hormones. Increases in prolactin levels following seizures, particularly if frequent, can interfere with the hypothalamic-pituitary-gonadal axis and affect ovulation. Diseases of limbic structure or function may well affect hypothalamic function. Finally, psychological and social development may be affected by epilepsy, particularly in those patients with intractable seizures starting early in life.

### 9.4 What preconception counselling should be given to women with epilepsy?

*The risk of teratogenesis is highest with polytherapy, and efforts should be made to reduce the number of drugs, to monotherapy if possible.* In a few patients with good seizure control, a doubtful diagnosis, or those taking prophylactic medication, it may prove possible to withdraw antiepileptic drugs altogether. However, if continuing antiepileptic drugs are necessary, the patient should be advised of the risks but reassured that the chance of serious congenital malformation is low. *Folate supplementation prior to pregnancy is recommended to try to minimise the risk of such malformations.*

**efforts to reduce drugs to monotherapy**

### 9.5 What is the effect of pregnancy on epilepsy?

In some women, pregnancy appears to have little effect on seizure frequency or severity, and in some, there is an improvement in seizure control. In about *one third of women with epilepsy who become pregnant, however, a deterioration in seizure control is experienced.* This may be due to several causes, including a fall in antiepileptic drug levels associated with physiological changes in pregnancy, as described below, poor compliance with the levels of antiepileptic drugs due to concern about teratogenesis, and, in some patients, sleep deprivation. In the first trimester, the high oestrogen:progesterone ratio may also play a part.

**deterioration in seizure control in some women**

### 9.6 Is there any special monitoring which needs to be carried out during pregnancy?

During the second and third trimester of pregnancy there is an increase of plasma volume of approximately one third, causing a dilutional effect and a consequent decrease in the level of antiepileptic drugs. However, the increase in plasma volume is not the entire explanation for the change in drug levels. In the case of phenytoin, the decline is maximal in the first trimester, while the decrease in carbamazepine levels is maximal in the third trimester. The level of valproate also falls, but in a more constant manner. Other explanations for the alteration in plasma levels include changes in clearance, differences in plasma protein binding and, rarely, diminished absorption.

**monitoring during pregnancy**

Because of these changes, it is advisable to see the patient regularly during pregnancy to keep a check on seizure control. *In patients who do not experience any change in seizure frequency, no specific changes are necessary*. In those with an increase in seizure frequency, it is helpful to monitor drug levels: because of the changes in plasma protein binding, free drug levels should be measured if possible. If a change in dosage of antiepileptic medication proves necessary, the pre-pregnancy dose of antiepileptic medication should be resumed at delivery.

**changes are not always necessary**

### 9.7 What is the risk of congenital malformations in the babies of women with epilepsy?

The most common congenital malformations in the babies of mothers taking antiepileptic drugs are cleft lip or palate (accounting for almost one third of the excess of malformations) and congenital heart defects, which occur in 1.5 to 2% of children, approximately three times that in the general population. Other major malformations include growth retardation, microcephaly, renal tube defects and learning difficulties. In addition a number of more minor anomalies, including hypertelorism, abnormalities of the epicanthal fold, short nose with broad nasal bridge, long upper lip, low-set ears, hirsutism, low hairline, distal digital hypoplasia, ptosis and V-shaped eyebrows, may occur. *Congenital malformations may be associated with all the commonly-used antiepileptic drugs, and although various syndromes have been described for specific drugs, the overlap is wide*. It is recommended that folate therapy 5 mg daily be given to all women with epilepsy before conception to minimise the risks of congenital malformation.

**the risk of defects**

**folate therapy can minimise the risks**

### 9.8 Are there any other problems specific to mothers with epilepsy?

Several studies suggest that women with epilepsy are at greater risk of obstetric complications, including vaginal bleeding, anaemia, hyperemesis gravidarum, and pre-eclampsia. Premature labour is more common than in women without epilepsy, and uterine contractions may be weak, so that intervention becomes necessary.

### 9.9 Should any particular problems be anticipated in the babies of mothers with epilepsy?

*The majority of women with epilepsy give birth to normal healthy infants.* Statistically there is a slight increase in perinatal problems, with a tendency towards lower Apgar scores, and an increased risk of difficult labour, asphyxia, prematurity and low birth weight. The risks of teratogenesis are discussed in Question 9.7. The risk of neonatal jaundice may be decreased as a result of hepatic enzyme induction by AEDs.

**normal, healthy infants**

### 9.10 Is it possible for patients taking antiepileptic drugs to breastfeed safely?

For the majority of women taking AEDs, breastfeeding may be undertaken without difficulty. AEDs are present in breast milk, at a concentration depending on the plasma protein binding (the more highly protein bound the drug, the lower the concentration in breast milk). Phenobarbitone and primidone (which is metabolised to phenobarbitone) sometimes cause problems with sedation, hypotonia and poor sucking, and occasionally it becomes necessary to stop breastfeeding on account of this. Jitteriness may occur in the baby on withdrawal of the drug. Hyperexcitability and poor sucking have also occasionally been reported with ethosuximide. Women taking acetazolamide or topiramate are advised not to breast feed.

**breast feeding and antiepileptic drugs**

### 9.11 What specific advice should be given to mothers with epilepsy who have young children?

Simple precautions should be taken by the mother with epilepsy when caring for her baby, particularly in the case of mothers having generalised tonic clonic seizures. Where there is the risk of dropping a baby, it is advisable to sit on floor cushions while feeding. For the same reason, washing and changing of the infant should take place on a waterproof mat placed on floor. It is recommended that someone else should be present in the house when the baby is bathed.

**care of babies and infants**

# CHAPTER 10

## PSYCHIATRY AND EPILEPSY

**10.1 What psychiatric disorders occur in people with epilepsy?**

There are three main categories of psychiatric disorders occurring in people with epilepsy. First, *the underlying cerebral lesion responsible for the epilepsy may also predispose to psychiatric changes*. This may be seen, for example, in patients with frontal lobe tumours, and in those with Alzheimer's disease. People with diffuse brain damage, who often have learning disabilities, are also prone to both seizures and psychiatric disorders.

*predisposition to psychiatric changes*

Secondly, *psychiatric disturbances may be directly associated with the seizures*. Prior to seizures, patients sometimes describe a prodrome in which they are tense, anxious, depressed or irritable. The ictus itself may also be associated with various abnormal experiences, among them psychosensory, affective, cognitive, and psychomotor symptoms. Psychosensory symptoms include illusions and hallucinations involving any sensory modality: for example, objects may appear to be increased in size (macropsia) or distorted. The most common ictal affective symptom is fear, but anger may occasionally occur. Pleasant ictal affective symptoms are described but are rare. Cognitive disturbances during seizures include dysmnestic symptoms such as déjà vu or jamais vu, forced thinking and feelings of unreality. Clouding of consciousness and psychomotor symptoms (automatisms) frequently occur during temporal lobe seizures. Automatisms often consist of chewing movements, fumbling with various objects or picking at clothes, and sometimes more complex activities such as undressing. They usually last only a few minutes, but on occasion may last longer.

*psychiatric disturbances and seizures*

*cognitive disturbances*

Occasionally ongoing epileptic activity may present as a confusional or obtunded state. This may occur in absence status, which occurs particularly in children, who appear confused, withdrawn and slow, sometimes alternating with period of relative normality. A few cases of absence status occurring de novo in adulthood have also been reported. Psychomotor status may also present as a confused state, sometimes accompanied by automatisms and occasionally with psychotic features.

Post-ictal psychiatric disorders are also relatively common. The majority of people will be confused and have some impairment of consciousness immediately after a seizure. However, some then go on to have a period of relative lucency, usually lasting one to two days, followed by a "post-ictal psychosis" in which they experience hallucinations and delusions, often paranoid in type. Such a psychosis may last for hours, days, or rarely even weeks. Treatment with such drugs as haloperidol may be necessary in the short term.

**confusion and impairment of consciousness**

Finally, *psychiatric disorders which are not related to seizure activity can occur in people with epilepsy, particularly those with seizures of temporal lobe origin.* These include personality disorders, affective disorders and psychoses. The arguments about the existence of an "epileptic personality" are discussed below. Behavioural problems occur in some children with epilepsy, and are often linked to overprotection by their parents, so that they become socially isolated and are emotionally immature and dependent. A number of studies have shown depression to be common in patients with epilepsy, particularly those in whom the onset of the condition occurs late in life. Often this is reactive, though endogenous depression may also occur. Suicide is five times more common in people with epilepsy than in the general population, and in people with temporal lobe epilepsy, it is 25 times more common. Anxiety is also common in people with epilepsy.

**psychiatric disorders in people with epilepsy**

*Psychoses are more common in people with epilepsy, particularly those with associated neurological deficits, than in the general population.* They particularly tend to occur in patients with long-standing, severe epilepsy, and are probably more prevalent in people with temporal lobe seizures, especially if a cerebral malformation (such as a hamartoma) is present. It has also been suggested that temporal lobe epilepsy associated with dysfunction of the left temporal lobe confers an increased risk of psychosis.

**psychoses in people with epilepsy**

Interictal psychoses occurring in people with epilepsy may be intermittent or chronic. There may be affective, paranoid or schizophrenia-like symptoms; commonly occurring features are paranoid, mystical and grandiose delusions, feelings of passivity, and auditory hallucinations. There is often better preservation of personality and affect than in schizophrenia.

Acute psychosis may also occur in association with certain antiepileptic drugs, and has been reported, for example, with vigabatrin and ethosuximide. This seems to occur more frequently in people with previous psychiatric illness, those with associated neurological deficits, and those in whom seizures cease abruptly following introduction of the drug.

### 10.2 What is the prevalence of psychiatric disorders in people with epilepsy?

Assessment of the prevalence of psychiatric morbidity in people with epilepsy depends to a great extent on the definitions used, both with regard to epilepsy (whether, for example, people having seizures at any time in the past should be included, or only those with active epilepsy or receiving treatment), and with regard to the definition of "psychiatric disorder". Partly because of the unpredictability of seizures, epilepsy itself is often a considerable source of stress, and anxiety and depression are particularly common in people with epilepsy. Studies of psychiatric morbidity may also suffer from selection bias as a result of the choice of population under study, since it has been shown that people with epilepsy who also have psychiatric disorders are more likely to be referred to hospital. Thus hospital-based studies are likely to give misleadingly high results. *Overall, the prevalence of psychiatric disorders in people with epilepsy seems to be of the order of 30-40%, although it may be as high as 60% in people with neurological deficits in addition to epilepsy.* Morbidity is also increased in people with temporal lobe seizure disorders. The prevalence of psychosis is much lower, with most studies giving figures of 1-3%, although some, mainly those studying hospital populations, give figures as high as 9%.

**the prevalence of psychiatric disorders**

### 10.3 What is "forced normalisation"?

"Forced normalisation" is a term which was originally used by Landolt to describe a state in which certain patients with seizures showing epileptic activity on the EEG, at other times developed a psychotic disturbance associated with a lack of electroencephalographic epileptic activity. The term "alternative psychosis" is also used to describe this psychosis occurring in association with normalisation of the EEG. Forced normalisation may occur either during spontaneous remission of seizures or as a result of treatment with antiepileptic drugs. It is not limited to

**describing forced normalisation and alternative psychosis**

patients with temporal lobe epilepsy, having also been reported not infrequently in patients with generalised epilepsies, although its overall occurrence is rare (less than 1% of patients with epilepsy).

### 10.4 Is there an "epileptic personality"?

**the debate over epileptic personalities**

Over the years there has been considerable debate as to whether an "epileptic personality" exists. Proponents of this view have suggested that certain characteristics are more commonly seen in people with epilepsy. Patients with temporal lobe epilepsy have been described as obsessional, circumstantial, "sticky", emotional, humourless, angry, suspicious, concrete, and having a preoccupation with religion and philosophy. Hyposexuality and hypergraphia have also been reported. Patients with juvenile myoclonic epilepsy, in contrast, have been described as having personality traits such as irresponsibility, quick temper, exaggeration and distractibility.

Although there are a number of factors which could explain an "epileptic personality", including the effect of medication, social isolation as a result of seizures, the stigma of epilepsy, and parental overprotection, and underlying brain damage, *the existence of a personality disorder in patients with epilepsy in the absence of such factors remains unproved*.

### 10.5 Can the memory be affected by epilepsy?

**Complaints of a poor memory are common**

*Complaints of a poor memory are very common in people with epilepsy, particularly those with temporal lobe seizures*. There are several factors which may be involved. In some instances, the underlying brain damage responsible for the epilepsy also causes memory impairment. In other patients, epileptic discharges occur frequently, and even though they may be insufficient to cause clinical seizures, they can interfere with memory function. Antiepileptic drugs are another possible cause of memory impairment, recognised with increasing frequency recently, although such problems are usually mild.

Despite the fact that many people with epilepsy do complain of memory problems, *psychological testing often does not support the presence of a major memory disturbance*. This may be because the tests used are not sensitive to subtle abnormalities of everyday memory function, but it may be that some patients are unduly anxious about minor memory abnormalities which are common in the general population.

### 10.6 What are pseudoseizures?

Pseudoseizures (also known as psychogenic seizures, hysterical seizures, or non-epileptic attack disorder (NEAD)) are *episodic disturbances which bear some resemblance to an epileptic seizure, but which do not have an epileptic cause*. Pseudoseizures are common, being the diagnosis in up to 20% of patients thought to have intractable seizures. They not infrequently occur in addition to epileptic seizures in people with epilepsy, but in recent years have been recognised increasingly in people without an epileptic disorder.

Pseudoseizures take many forms (for example convulsion, swoon, altered behaviour), and have a variety of different causes. They may represent a misinterpretation of such symptoms as dizziness or anxiety (which may themselves be physiological or pathological). *Most commonly they have a psychological cause*, often an anxiety neurosis although occasionally they may occur in the context of a psychosis. Although pseudoseizures often take the form of a layman's image of an epileptic attack, they are usually not consciously simulated.

**pseudoseizures have a psychological cause**

*Diagnosis may be difficult, particularly since some genuine epileptic seizures, especially those of frontal lobe origin, may have a bizarre appearance*. However, it is often possible to distinguish pseudoseizures on a clinical basis if one is witnessed, or recorded using prolonged EEG-video monitoring. The onset of pseudoseizures is often gradual, sometimes occurring in response to suggestion or the presence of others in the room. Initial cyanosis does not occur. Jerking of limbs is usually less rhythmical than is the case in epileptic seizures, often taking the form of wild asynchronous thrashing movements. Tongue-biting and incontinence may occur, but are less common than in epileptic seizures. Attempts to open the patient's eyes are often forcibly resisted. Post-ictal drowsiness or confusion is uncommon, and the widespread slowing seen on EEG after a generalised tonic clonic seizure is usually absent. Measurement of serum prolactin levels in the post-ictal phase may be helpful in the distinction between convulsive pseudoseizures and generalised tonic clonic seizures, although it is less consistently useful in the diagnosis of more minor attacks. *Pseudoseizures are refractory to antiepileptic medication, and a lack of response may be the first indication of this diagnosis in some patients.*

**distinguishing between epileptic and pseudoseizures**

### 10.7 How should pseudoseizures be treated?

The treatment of pseudoseizures depends on the underlying cause, and may be complicated and difficult. If the diagnosis is the result of misinterpretation of symptoms, advice and reassurance may suffice. If the pseudoseizures are the result of more complex psychological problems, the underlying issues need to be examined closely and the help of a psychiatrist enlisted. It is rarely helpful in such cases to confront the patient with "putting on seizures" or reject him or her for the same reason; rather, a positive approach should be taken in which the attacks are recognised as a real problem, but treatment directed at the underlying disturbance.

### Reference

Trimble MR, Ring HA. Psychological and Psychiatric aspects of Epilepsy.
In: Clinical Epilepsy. Duncan JS, Shorvon SD, Fish DR. Edinburgh: Churchill Livingstone, 1995: 321-348.

Trimble MR. Psychiatric Disorders in Epilespsy.
In: The treatment of Epilepsy. Shorvon SD, Dreifuss F, Fish DR, Thomas D (eds.). Oxford: Blackwell 1996: 337-344.

# CHAPTER 11

## GENETIC COUNSELLING

### 11.1 To what extent does genetic inheritance play a part in the development of epilepsy?

It has long been recognised that epilepsy has a genetic component, and that this is considerably greater in idiopathic than symptomatic epilepsy. A genetic predisposition is also indicated by the fact that many well recognised genetically-determined neurological disorders (such as tuberous sclerosis, fragile X syndrome, Angelman syndrome, and the mitochondrial encephalopathies) are associated with epilepsy.

*It is likely that many forms of epilepsy have multifactorial (polygenic) inheritance.* However, in recent years gene mapping has been accomplished in three specific epilepsy syndromes: benign familial neonatal convulsions (long arm of chromosome 20), juvenile myoclonic epilepsy (JME) (short arm of chromosome 6) and the Unverricht-Lundborg form of progressive myoclonus epilepsy (long arm of chromosome 21). Benign familial neonatal convulsions are inherited in an autosomal dominant manner with a penetrance of 85%. Unverricht-Lundborg disease is inherited as an autosomal recessive condition, while the inheritance of JME continues to be debated.

**genetic factors affecting epilepsy**

### 11.2 What is the risk of a patient with epilepsy having a child with epilepsy?

In view of the above, this clearly depends on the type of epilepsy. It is also affected by a number of other factors, for example, the sex of the parent with epilepsy (the risk being greater when the mother is affected), the age at which the parent developed epilepsy (the risk being greater if this was at a young age), the occurrence of epilepsy in the other parent or another sibling, and the presence of EEG abnormalities in the child at risk. Figure 23 summarises these risks. *Genetic counselling may be helpful in quantifying the risks more precisely for an individual.*

**quantifying the genetic risks**

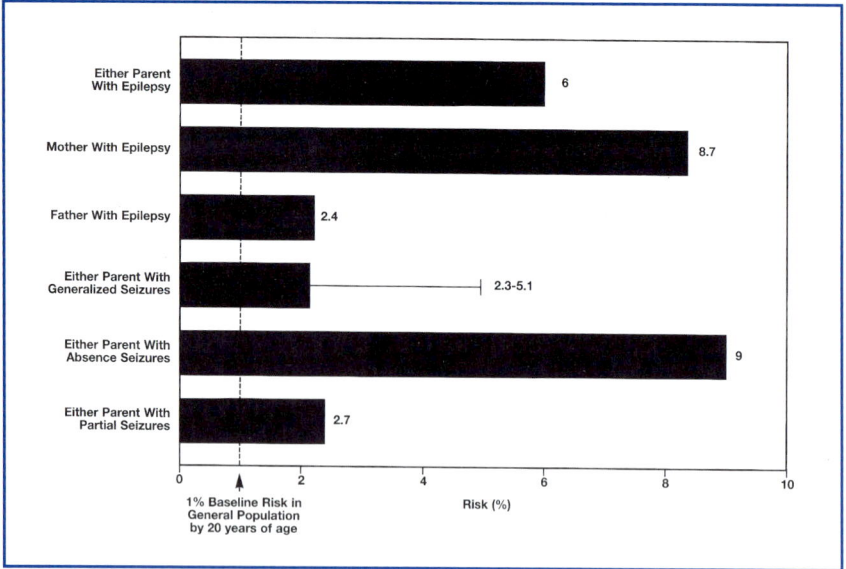

**Figure 23.** *Diagram showing risk of an epileptic patient bearing a child with epilepsy. Reproduced with permission from: Hauser WA, Hesdorffer DC. Facts about Epilepsy. Landover, Epilepsy Foundation of America, 1990.*

### 11.3 What is the chance of epilepsy developing in the sibling of a person with epilepsy?

**sibling development**

Again, this depends on the type of epilepsy and other factors including age at onset and whether more than one family member is affected. Studies of children with generalised epilepsy have estimated the risk of epilepsy developing in siblings at about 4-8% (and of any non-febrile seizures at 6-12%), although almost 50% may show generalised spike and wave abnormalities on their EEG at some time. The risk is increased if a parent is also affected. For most patients with seizures of partial origin the risk of non-febrile seizures developing in siblings is about 3-5% by the age of 40 years. However, the chance of seizures developing is considerably greater (about 15%) in siblings of children with benign childhood epilepsy with centrotemporal spikes.

### 11.4 What percentage of babies born to patients with epilepsy have significant congenital abnormalities?

Most estimates of the proportion of babies having significant congenital malformations born to patients *with epilepsy range from around 4 to 10%,* although a few studies have found the rate to be as high as 16 to 18%. This compares with a malformation rate of about 2 to 3% in the general population.

**congenital malformations in babies**

### 11.5 What are the principal causes of these?

There are several possible mechanisms. These include the facts that the epilepsy itself may be secondary to a genetic abnormality, and that anoxic or other damage may occur during seizures while the foetus is in utero. However, by far the majority of malformations are thought to be associated with the use of antiepileptic drugs by the mother during pregnancy, the "foetal antiepileptic drug syndrome". The risk is increased by the use of polytherapy, but the influence of serum drug concentrations on the risk of congenital anomalies remains controversial. There is a slight increase in the risk of malformations in the children born to fathers taking antiepileptic therapy.

**causes and risks of abnormalities**

E PILEPSY

# CHAPTER 12

## WORK, LEISURE AND EPILEPSY

### 12.1 How does epilepsy affect a child's education?

In many countries recent government policies have encouraged a shift towards including people with disabilities in mainstream schooling, rather than advocating the provision of special schools. *In the UK the majority of children with epilepsy are now integrated into mainstream schools*, while most of those still being educated in special schools are there because of associated handicaps. Factors which may affect the educational performance of the child with epilepsy include such handicaps as well as the effect of medication, the effect of subclinical seizure discharges causing lapses in concentration or other cognitive impairment, and time off school as a result of epilepsy. Social isolation as a result of overprotection, problems caused by overindulgence, and the low expectations of parents and teachers may complicate the situation. *The child should be encouraged to participate in almost all school activities and sports, with the possible exception of climbing.*

**children with epilepsy in the mainstream classroom**

### 12.2 How does epilepsy affect a person's prospects of employment?

Many studies have found an increased rate of unemployment or underemployment among people with epilepsy. This has been attributed to several factors. The seizures themselves may render certain types of employment (particularly where driving is involved) unsuitable; associated handicaps may also limit the choice of work. People with epilepsy may lack educational qualifications if they have missed a large amount of schooling, while parental overprotection may cause isolation and poor social adaptation. It seems probable, however, that the stigma of epilepsy has been responsible for a significant proportion of unemployment and underemployment, often because of a poor understanding about epilepsy or worries about public image, safety or insurance.

**epilepsy in the workplace**

## 12.3 Are there any jobs which cannot be performed by a person with epilepsy?

People with epilepsy are limited from holding posts in which driving is a necessity by the law prevailing in the particular country or state. The laws regarding the driving of passenger vehicles or heavy goods vehicles are usually stricter. Other areas of employment in which statutory barriers to the employment of people with epilepsy may be present are the police force, fire brigade, armed services and merchant navy, teaching, and the prison, coastguard, and ambulance services. Types of work which could pose particular hazards for people with epilepsy include work with unguarded machinery, work near tanks of water or chemicals, and work with valuable fragile objects.

**potential job hazards**

Where there are no statutory barriers, the type and severity of a person's epilepsy, the degree of seizure control, and the presence of associated handicaps are all important in assessing the suitability of a particular type of employment.

## 12.4 Does a person with epilepsy have to declare the condition when he or she applies for a job?

A dilemma may arise for the person with epilepsy applying for work if he feels that his seizures may present an obstacle to his obtaining the job. Failure to disclose the diagnosis can mean that the employer's insurance cover is invalidated. Provided that the epilepsy is disclosed and the employee is in a suitable job, most employers' insurance policies do not discriminate against disabled people. Where a prospective employee is required to complete a pre-employment health questionnaire, concealing the diagnosis may render the employee subject to dismissal and unable to claim that the dismissal was unfair at an industrial tribunal. However, to prevent the possibility of discrimination on account of one's health it is becoming increasingly common for such information to be disclosed only to the occupational health physician after recommendation for employment. The practices of individual companies may vary, but provided that the epilepsy does not constitute a bar to employment for safety reasons, it should usually only be necessary for the occupational health physician, and the employee's immediate supervisor in the case of active epilepsy, to know about the diagnosis.

**employment regulations for people with epilepsy**

### 12.5 Can people with epilepsy safely do shift work?

There has been little research into this aspect of employment. Issues of concern when people with epilepsy do shift work are that they should obtain adequate sleep, and that they should take their medication regularly to avoid the risk of withdrawal seizures or seizures occurring during drowsiness. It has been reported that few problems have been encountered when these conditions have been met.

**additional job safety concerns**

### 12.6 What restrictions on leisure activity should be placed on the person with epilepsy?

The risk of injury as a result of leisure activities depends partly on the type and frequency of seizures. *In general, the person with epilepsy should try to lead as normal and unrestricted a life as possible*; considerable psychological damage may occur as a result of overprotection. However, it is important to take simple precautions to try to minimise the risk of injury if seizures causing loss of consciousness should occur, and simple advice such as avoiding unguarded heights and not standing on the edge of station platforms, reservoirs and so on should be given. Participation in most sports is possible, even by people continuing to have seizures, although sub aqua diving, caving, and contact sports such as wrestling and boxing should be avoided. *Swimming and riding are acceptable provided the person with epilepsy is accompanied by someone aware of the seizures who could help if necessary.*

**leading a normal life**

### 12.7 What is the law regarding driving by people who have had seizures?

The law with respect to driving by people with seizures differs from country to country, and within the United States, from state to state. Most countries demand a period of seizure-freedom of one or two years before a licence is granted, although in some the period is shorter or longer. The importance of seizure-type also varies; in some patients any type of seizure will cause loss of the driving licence, while in others patients experiencing only simple partial seizures or myoclonic jerks are permitted to drive. The laws regarding the driving of heavy goods vehicles are usually stricter.

**driving limitations**

**12.8 Does the law require a doctor to inform the licensing authority that his patient has epilepsy?**

Again, this varies from country to country. In some the onus is on the patient, while in others, the doctor is responsible for informing the licensing authority about a diagnosis of epilepsy in one of his patients.

**12.9 Does epilepsy have other legal implications?**

**important legal issues**

Because of the nature of epilepsy, and in particular the fact that during both the ictal and post-ictal phases "automatic", subconscious, behaviour may occur, it is occasionally claimed that crimes have been committed during the course of a seizure. Certain criteria should be fulfilled before an epileptic automatism can be held responsible. The person should be known to have epilepsy, there should be no premeditation, the offence should be inappropriate and out of character for the patient, and the patient should have impaired consciousness at the time of the offence, together with amnesia for the event. Although the prevalence of epilepsy among prisoners is considerably higher than in the general population, it is very rare for crimes to be committed during a seizure, and the increased prevalence can be explained on the basis of organic brain damage leading to impaired capacity, aggression and antisocial behaviour.

# CHAPTER 13

## QUESTIONS PATIENTS MAY ASK ABOUT EPILEPSY

The following questions are those most commonly asked of the information service run by a voluntary organisation for people with epilepsy. A brief answer is given in each case, together with the appropriate reference.

### 13.1 Where can I get some general literature on epilepsy?

A list of organisations able to provide such information is given in Appendix 2.

### 13.2 I have just been diagnosed as having epilepsy and want to know what I can or cannot do

People with epilepsy should try to lead as normal a life as possible. There are, however, some sensible precautions which should be taken to avoid **quality of life** injury in the case of seizures. These are discussed more fully in Chapter 12: they include swimming only when accompanied, and the avoidance of unguarded heights, water, and fires. There are also restrictions on driving in patients with uncontrolled epilepsy, and certain professions are barred to people with epilepsy. It is important to advise each patient individually, taking into account the nature of his or her seizures.

### 13.3 I have just been diagnosed with epilepsy and want to know if I will have it for the rest of my life.

The majority (60-70%) of people developing seizures enter long-term **looking at the** remission, usually soon after starting medication, and in about 50% it is **future** eventually possible for medication to be discontinued without recurrence of seizures. In a few people, especially those with such conditions as West syndrome and Lennox-Gastaut syndrome, seizures are more difficult to control (see Chapters 3 and 7).

### 13.4 Who do I have to tell that I have epilepsy?

**informing the relevant people**

It is advisable for people with epilepsy, particularly if poorly controlled, to inform their colleagues at work or teachers at school, so that appropriate measures may be taken in the event of seizures. It is also wise for patients to carry a card or wear a bracelet or medallion advising about their medical condition. Prospective employers may ask about medical conditions, and disclosure of epilepsy is advisable, even though this may cause some problems for persons seeking employment. The International Bureau for Epilepsy has issued guidelines for employers, "Employing people with epilepsy: principles for good practice" which can be obtained from their local branches or from their headquarters, International Bureau for Epilepsy, PO Box 21, 2100 AA Heemstede, the Netherlands.

### 13.5 Do the drugs that I take for my epilepsy have side-effects?

**treatment questions**

All drugs have the potential to cause adverse effects in some people, as detailed in Chapter 7. However, if these do occur, they are often mild, and most people are able to take antiepileptic drugs with few if any problems.

### 13.6 Is there any alternative to taking anti epileptic drugs?

People who have very mild or infrequent seizures, or only nocturnal attacks, may not need to take medication. Those having seizures only with known precipitants may also be able to manage simply by avoiding the triggering factors. However, in most people drug treatment is necessary, at least for a period of time. Surgery may be helpful in a small proportion of people who have not responded fully to antiepileptic drugs, but medication usually needs to be continued afterwards.

### 13.7 Will the drugs that I take affect my having children?

**concerns about pregnancy**

There is a small increase in the risk of congenital abnormalities in the offspring of people with epilepsy, in part attributable to medication (see Chapter 9). However, the risk from uncontrolled seizures is greater in most women than the risk of continuing antiepileptic medication during pregnancy.

**13.8 My young daughter who has epilepsy has been told that she may not take part in some of the activities, such as swimming as the other children. Is this really necessary?**

Most school activities, including swimming, can be undertaken by children with epilepsy, provided that supervision is adequate. If seizures are uncontrolled, it is advised that the child avoids climbing activities (see Chapter 12).

**children and sports**

**13.9 How long do I have to surrender my driving licence if I have only minor seizures and do not lose consciousness during my seizures?**

The laws governing driving vary in different countries, both with regard to the need to surrender the licence if consciousness is not lost during seizures, and the length of time for which driving is not permitted. It is advisable to check with the appropriate authority in each case.

**driving and the law**

**13.10 How can I get in touch with other people who have epilepsy who could tell me about problems they may well have experienced and overcome?**

A list of national voluntary organisations is given in the Appendix A. They are usually able to supply the addresses of local support groups for people with epilepsy. It is advisable for the physician looking after people with epilepsy to have a list of the local organisations.

**epilepsy support groups**

**13.11 Can you give me any information about how to manage different types of seizures?**

The acute management of generalised tonic clonic seizures is given in Chapter 7. The majority of seizures are self-limited, and no specific management is required apart from ensuring safety and reassuring the patient when the seizure is over.

**management of seizures**

**13.12 My husband and I would like to start a family, but I have epilepsy. Will our children develop epilepsy?**

For the majority of people with epilepsy, the chance of a child developing epilepsy is very small (Chapter 11). It is slightly higher in some specific epilepsy syndromes, such as the generalised idiopathic epilepsies.

**genetic concerns**

**13.13 I have two children. The elder did not have the whooping cough vaccine as my sister has epilepsy. Now I am being advised to have my younger one vaccinated. What should I do?**

**vaccination fears in children**

Although in the past it was advised that relatives of people with epilepsy should not be vaccinated, this advice has now been superseded (see Chapter 4).

**13.14 I have had quite severe seizures for many years and the drugs do not seem to help. Could I be helped with surgery?**

**an alternative to medication**

A proportion of people with seizures intractable to medical treatment may be helped with surgery. This is particularly the case for people with temporal lobe seizures. This is discussed in more detail in Chapter 8.

**13.15 I had what doctors think were three seizures over the past six months but the EEG and CT scan were normal. However, I am still being diagnosed as having epilepsy - why?**

**investigation of seizures**

Although the EEG and CT may show abnormalities in people with epilepsy, it is not at all uncommon for them to be normal. This is because epilepsy is an episodic disorder of neuronal function, i.e. in between attacks both the examination of the patient, and investigations may be unremarkable (see Chapter 6).

# APPENDIX 1

## FURTHER READING

Aicardi J. Epilepsy in Children. New York: Raven Press 1994.

Engel Jr., Jerome. Seizures and Epilepsy. Philadelphia: F.A. Davis 1989.

Engel Jr., Jerome (ed.). Surgical Treatment of Epilepsy. Second edition; New York: Raven Press 1993.

Dam, Mogens; Gram, Lennart (eds.). Comprehensive Epileptology. New York: Raven Press 1991.

Duncan JS, Panayiotopoulos CP (eds). The typical absences and related epileptic syndromes. Edinburgh: Churchill Livingstone; 1994.

Duncan JS, Shorvon SD, Fish DR. Clinical Epilepsy. Edinburgh: Churchill Livingstone; 1995.

Hauser WA, Hesdorffer DH. Epilepsy: frequency, causes and consequences. New York: Demos Press, 1990.

Hopkins A, Shorvon SD, Cascino G. Epilepsy. London: Chapman & Hall 1995.

Laidlaw J, Richens A, Chadwick D (eds.). A textbook of epilepsy. Fourth edition; Edinburgh: Churchill Livingstone, 1993.

Levy RH, Mattson R, Meldrum BS. Antiepileptic Drugs. New York: Raven Press, 1995.

Roger J, Bureau M, Dravet C et al. (eds.). Epileptic Syndromes in Infancy, Childhood and Adolescence. London: John Libbey 1992.

Shorvon SD, Dreifuss FE, Fish DR, Thomas DGT. The treatment of epilepsy. Oxford: Blackwell; 1996.

Shorvon SD. Status epilepticus: clinical features and treatment in children and adults. Cambridge: University Press 1994.

Wyllie E (ed.). The treatment of epilepsy: Principles and practice. Philadelphia/London: Lea and Febiger, 1993.

# APPENDIX 2

## EPILEPSY ORGANISATIONS AND OTHER USEFUL ADDRESSES

The International League Against Epilepsy (ILAE) is an international organisation for medical and paramedical professionals involved in the care of people with epilepsy. It has branches in over 50 countries. Details of local branches can be obtained from: Professor Simon Shorvon, Vice-President, ILAE,

Chalfont Centre for Epilepsy
Chalfont St Peter
Buckinghamshire  SL9 ORJ
England.

The International Bureau for Epilepsy (IBE) is an international voluntary organisation for people with epilepsy and their friends and carers. It has branches and affiliated societies in many countries, some of which have been kindly supplied by The International Bureau for Epilepsy and listed below.

### IBE HEADQUARTERS

P.O. Box 21
2100 AA Heemstede
Holland

### ARGENTINA

Ass. de Lucha contra la Epilepsia
Tucuman 3261
1425 Buenos Aires

### AUSTRALIA

National Epilepsy Association of Australia
P.O. Box 224
Parramatta NSW 2150

## AUSTRIA

Epilepsie Selbsthilfegruppen Österreichs
Hauptstr. 44/2/2
2344 Ma. Enzersdorf

## BELGIUM

Belg. Nat. Bond tegen Epilepsie
Avenue Albert 135
Brussels 1060

## BRAZIL

Assoc. Brasileira de Epilepsia
UNICAMP - Cx. Postal: 6138
13.081-970 Campinas SP

## CAMEROON

Epilespy Research and Action Center (ERAC)
P.O. Box 14606
Yaounde

## CANADA

Mrs. Denise Crepin
Epilepsy Canada
1470 Peel Street, suite 745
Montreal, Quebec H3A 1T1

## CHILE

Ass. Liga contra la Epilepsia de Valparaiso
P.O. Box 705
Vina del Mar

## COLOMBIA

Liga Colombiana contra la Epilepsia
P.O. Box 057751
Bogota DC

**CUBA**

Capitulo Cubano BIE
Instituto de Neurologia y Neurocirugia
29y D, Vedado
C. de la Habana, 42

**CZECH REPUBLIC**

Spolecnost "E"
Novodvorská 994
142 21 Praha 4

**DENMARK**

Dansk Epilepsiforening
Dr. Sellsvej 28
DK 4293 Dianalund

**ECUADOR**

Asoc. de Padres de Niños con Epilepsia
Isla Marchena 300 y Los Granados
P.O. Box 17-15-221 C
Quito

Liga Tung. de Control de la Epilepsia
Mera 5-27 y Sucre
Segundo Piso, Ambato

**FINLAND**

Mrs. Leena Hyvärinen
Epilepsyaliitto
Kalevankatu 61
00180 Helsinki 18

**FRANCE**

Mrs. Jacqueline Beaussart-Defaye
A.I.S.P.A.C.E.
11 Avenue Kennedy
F-59800 Lille

Mrs. Brigitte Bonard-Braeck
Bureau Français de l'Épilepsie
236 bis, rue de Tolbiac
75013 Paris

**GERMANY**

Mr. Robert Bauer
Deutsche Epilepsie Vereinigung
Zillestrasse 102
10585 Berlin

**GREECE**

Dr. A. Covanis
Greek National Association against Epilepsy
Aghia Sophia Children's Hospital, dept. of Neur./Neurophys
Athens 11527

**GUATEMALA**

Dr. Henry B. Stokes
Guatemalan Epilepsy Society, CAGUALICE
Av. La Reforma 1-64, Zona 9
Guatemala Ciudad

**ICELAND**

The Epilepsy Association of Iceland
Postbox 5182
126 Reykjavík

## INDIA

Indian Epilepsy Association
nr. 1 Old Veterinary Hospital Road
Basavanagudi Bangalore 560 004

## INDONESIA

Yayasan Epilepsi Indonesia
Jl. Senayan No. 16, Block S
Kebayoran Baru, Jakarta
Selatan 12180

PERPEI
JL. Jelita Utara no. 11, Rawamangun
Jakarta 13220

## IRELAND

Irish Epilepsy Association
249 Crumlin Road
Dublin 12

## ISRAEL

Israel Epilepsy Association
4 Avodat Yisrael St.
P.O. Box 1598
Jerusalem

Mr. Yaacov Nir
Association of Epileptics in Israel
P.O. Box 5355
Herzlia 46101

## ITALY

Mrs. Raffaella Rizzo
Associazione Italiana contro l'Epilessia (AICE)
Via Copernico 28
40058 Malalbergo (BO)

## JAPAN

Dr. T. Soga
Epilepsy Hospital Bethel
27-4 Hata-Mukaiyama Kitahase
Iwanuma-City 989-24

Dr. M. Seino
National Epilepsy Center
Shizuoka Higashi Hospital
886 Urushiyama
Shizuoka 420

The Japanese Epilepsy Association
5F Zenkokuzaidan Building 2-2-8
Nishiwaseda Shinjuku - Ku
Tokyo 162

## KENYA

Mrs. Caroline Pickering
Kenya Association f/t Welfare of Epileptics
P.O. Box 60790
Nairobi

## KOREA

Korean Epilepsy Association/Rose Club
#110-021, Room no.301
BuwonBld., 175-1 Buam-dong
Chongno-Ku
Seoul

Chairman Songpo Epilepsy Foundation Korea
#302 Dongil B/D, 170 Insadong
Chongro-Ku
Seoul, 110-290

## MEXICO

Group Acceptation de Epilepticos
Amsterdam 1928 # 19
Colonia Olimpica-Pedregal
Mexico 04710 D.F.

## NEW ZEALAND

Epilepsy Association of New Zealand Inc.
P.O. Box 1074
Hamilton

## NORWAY

Norsk Epilepsiforbund
Storgt. 39
0182 Oslo

## POLAND

Polish Epilepsy Association
15-482 Bialystok
Ul. Fabryczna 57 (XIp. pok.7)

## PORTUGAL

Liga Nac. Portug. c.l. Epilepsia
Rua Sá da Bandeira 162-1 piso
4000 Porto

## SLOVENIA

Liga Proti Epilepsiji
CIPD, Njegoseva 4/11
61 000 Ljubljana

## SOUTH AFRICA

South African National Epilepsy League, S.A.N.E.L.
P. O. Box 73
Observatory 7935

## SPAIN

P.E.N.E.P.A.
Calle Escuelas Pias n. 89
Barcelona 08017

**SRI LANKA**

Epilepsy Association of Sri Lanka
10 Austin Place
Colombo 8

**SWEDEN**

Swedish Epilepsy Association
P.O. Box 9514
10274 Stockholm

**SWITZERLAND**

Prof. Dr. P.A. Despland
Swiss League against Epilepsy
Feldeggstrasse 71, P.O. Box 1332
8032 Zurich

Mrs. Regina M. Henggeler
ParEpi Geschäftstelle
Waldhofstrasse 21
6314 Unterägeri

Dr. Chr. Pachlatko
Swiss Epilepsy Centre
Bleulerstrasse 60
CH-8008 Zürich

**THE NETHERLANDS**

Mevr. E. Groeneweg
Dr. Hans Berger Kliniek
Postbus 90108
4800 RA Breda

Mrs. Marijke de Puit
Epilepsie Vereniging Nederland
P.O. Box 270
3990 GB Houten

The Director, Instituut voor Epilepsiebestrijding
Meer & Bosch/Cruquiushoeve
P.O. Box 21
2100 AA Heemstede

Mr. C. Vroon
National Epilepsie Fonds/De Macht van het Kleine
Postbue 270
3990 GB Houten

Stichting Kempenhaeghe
Sterkselseweg 65
5591 VE Heeze

## U.K.

Mr. Gerald Chew
St. Piers Lingfield
St. Piers Lane
Lingfield
Surrey  RH7 6NG

Mr. Philip Lee
British Epilepsy Association
Anstey House
40 Hanover Square
Leeds LS3 1BE

David Lewis
Centre for Epilepsy
Warford, Near Alderley Edge
Cheshire SK9 7UD

National Society for Epilepsy Chalfont
Chalfont St. Peter
Gerrards Cross
Buckingamshire SL9 ORJ

Mrs. Lynn Sheldon
Gravesend Epilepsy Network
13 St. George's Crescent
Gravesend
Kent DA 12 4AR

Mrs. Judy Cochrane
Epilepsy Association of Scotland
48 Govan Road
Glasgow G51 1JL
Scotland

Mrs. Karen Jackson
Enlighten, Action for Epilepsy
Edinburgh, Mid & East Lothian
5 Coates Place
Edinburgh EH3 7AA
Scotland

Epilespi Cymru - Epilepsy Wales
Y Pant Teg, Brynteg
Dolgellau LL40 1RP Gwynedd
Wales

**U.S.A.**

Epilepsy Foundation of America
4351 Garden City Drive
Landover Maryland 20785

**ZIMBABWE**

Epilepsy Support Foundation
P.O. Box A104 Avondale
Old General Hospital
Mazoe Street
Harare

# INDEX

# QUESTIONS GUIDE

**Chapter 1**

Q1.1    Definition of epilepsy and epileptic seizures


**Chapter 2**

Q2.1    Classification of seizures

Q2.2    Partial seizures

Q2.3    Sub-divided partial seizures

Q2.4    Generalised seizures

Q2.5    Classification of epileptic syndromes

Q2.6    Characteristics of the main epileptic syndromes

Q2.7    Precipitating factors leading to seizures

Q2.8    Nocturnal seizures

Q2.9    Status epilepticus

Q2.10   The features of tonic clonic status epilepticus

Q2.11   The manifestations of non-convulsive status epilepticus

Q2.12   Absence status

Q2.13   Features of atypical absence status

Q2.14   Presentation of complex partial status epilepticus


**Chapter 3**

Q3.1    Difficulties of studying the epidemiology of epilepsy

Q3.2    The incidence of epilepsy

Q3.3    The prevalence of epilepsy

Q3.4    The prognosis of epilepsy

Q3.5    The risk of recurrence after a first epileptic attack

Q3.6    The risk of seizure recurrence after discontinuing anti epileptic treatment

Q3.7    The mortality of epilepsy

Q3.8    The risks of death from epilepsy

Q3.9    Causes of death in those with epilepsy


**Chapter 4**

Q4.1    Definition of (epileptic/threshold)

Q4.2    Most common aetiologies of epilepsy

Q4.3    Most common genetically determined epilepsies

## Chapter 5

E PILEPSY